Military instructions: including each particular motion of the manual and platoon exercises; elucidated with very minute drawings by Mr. R. K. Porter; ... By David Roberts, ...

David Roberts

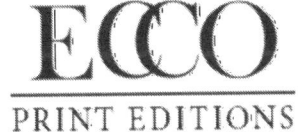

ECCO
PRINT EDITIONS

Military instructions: including each particular motion of the manual and platoon exercises;
elucidated with very minute drawings by Mr. R. K. Porter; ... By David Roberts, ...
Roberts, David
ESTCID: T112516
Reproduction from British Library
With a half-title.
London : printed for T. Egerton, 1798.
[8],36p.,plates ; 4°

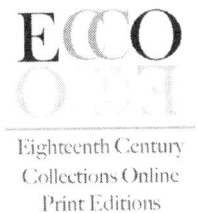

Gale ECCO Print Editions

Relive history with *Eighteenth Century Collections Online*, now available in print for the independent historian and collector. This series includes the most significant English-language and foreign-language works printed in Great Britain during the eighteenth century, and is organized in seven different subject areas including literature and language; medicine, science, and technology; and religion and philosophy. The collection also includes thousands of important works from the Americas.

The eighteenth century has been called "The Age of Enlightenment." It was a period of rapid advance in print culture and publishing, in world exploration, and in the rapid growth of science and technology – all of which had a profound impact on the political and cultural landscape. At the end of the century the American Revolution, French Revolution and Industrial Revolution, perhaps three of the most significant events in modern history, set in motion developments that eventually dominated world political, economic, and social life.

In a groundbreaking effort, Gale initiated a revolution of its own: digitization of epic proportions to preserve these invaluable works in the largest online archive of its kind. Contributions from major world libraries constitute over 175,000 original printed works. Scanned images of the actual pages, rather than transcriptions, recreate the works *as they first appeared.*

Now for the first time, these high-quality digital scans of original works are available via print-on-demand, making them readily accessible to libraries, students, independent scholars, and readers of all ages.

For our initial release we have created seven robust collections to form one the world's most comprehensive catalogs of 18th century works.

Initial Gale ECCO Print Editions collections include:

History and Geography
Rich in titles on English life and social history, this collection spans the world as it was known to eighteenth-century historians and explorers. Titles include a wealth of travel accounts and diaries, histories of nations from throughout the world, and maps and charts of a world that was still being discovered. Students of the War of American Independence will find fascinating accounts from the British side of conflict.

Social Science

Delve into what it was like to live during the eighteenth century by reading the first-hand accounts of everyday people, including city dwellers and farmers, businessmen and bankers, artisans and merchants, artists and their patrons, politicians and their constituents. Original texts make the American, French, and Industrial revolutions vividly contemporary.

Medicine, Science and Technology

Medical theory and practice of the 1700s developed rapidly, as is evidenced by the extensive collection, which includes descriptions of diseases, their conditions, and treatments. Books on science and technology, agriculture, military technology, natural philosophy, even cookbooks, are all contained here.

Literature and Language

Western literary study flows out of eighteenth-century works by Alexander Pope, Daniel Defoe, Henry Fielding, Frances Burney, Denis Diderot, Johann Gottfried Herder, Johann Wolfgang von Goethe, and others. Experience the birth of the modern novel, or compare the development of language using dictionaries and grammar discourses.

Religion and Philosophy

The Age of Enlightenment profoundly enriched religious and philosophical understanding and continues to influence present-day thinking. Works collected here include masterpieces by David Hume, Immanuel Kant, and Jean-Jacques Rousseau, as well as religious sermons and moral debates on the issues of the day, such as the slave trade. The Age of Reason saw conflict between Protestantism and Catholicism transformed into one between faith and logic -- a debate that continues in the twenty-first century.

Law and Reference

This collection reveals the history of English common law and Empire law in a vastly changing world of British expansion. Dominating the legal field is the *Commentaries of the Law of England* by Sir William Blackstone, which first appeared in 1765. Reference works such as almanacs and catalogues continue to educate us by revealing the day-to-day workings of society.

Fine Arts

The eighteenth-century fascination with Greek and Roman antiquity followed the systematic excavation of the ruins at Pompeii and Herculaneum in southern Italy; and after 1750 a neoclassical style dominated all artistic fields. The titles here trace developments in mostly English-language works on painting, sculpture, architecture, music, theater, and other disciplines. Instructional works on musical instruments, catalogs of art objects, comic operas, and more are also included.

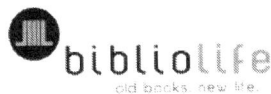

The BiblioLife Network

This project was made possible in part by the BiblioLife Network (BLN), a project aimed at addressing some of the huge challenges facing book preservationists around the world. The BLN includes libraries, library networks, archives, subject matter experts, online communities and library service providers. We believe every book ever published should be available as a high-quality print reproduction; printed on-demand anywhere in the world. This insures the ongoing accessibility of the content and helps generate sustainable revenue for the libraries and organizations that work to preserve these important materials.

The following book is in the "public domain" and represents an authentic reproduction of the text as printed by the original publisher. While we have attempted to accurately maintain the integrity of the original work, there are sometimes problems with the original work or the micro-film from which the books were digitized. This can result in minor errors in reproduction. Possible imperfections include missing and blurred pages, poor pictures, markings and other reproduction issues beyond our control. Because this work is culturally important, we have made it available as part of our commitment to protecting, preserving, and promoting the world's literature.

GUIDE TO FOLD-OUTS MAPS and OVERSIZED IMAGES

The book you are reading was digitized from microfilm captured over the past thirty to forty years. Years after the creation of the original microfilm, the book was converted to digital files and made available in an online database.

In an online database, page images do not need to conform to the size restrictions found in a printed book. When converting these images back into a printed bound book, the page sizes are standardized in ways that maintain the detail of the original. For large images, such as fold-out maps, the original page image is split into two or more pages

Guidelines used to determine how to split the page image follows:

• Some images are split vertically; large images require vertical and horizontal splits.
• For horizontal splits, the content is split left to right.
• For vertical splits, the content is split from top to bottom.
• For both vertical and horizontal splits, the image is processed from top left to bottom right.

MILITARY INSTRUCTIONS.

FRONTISPIECE.

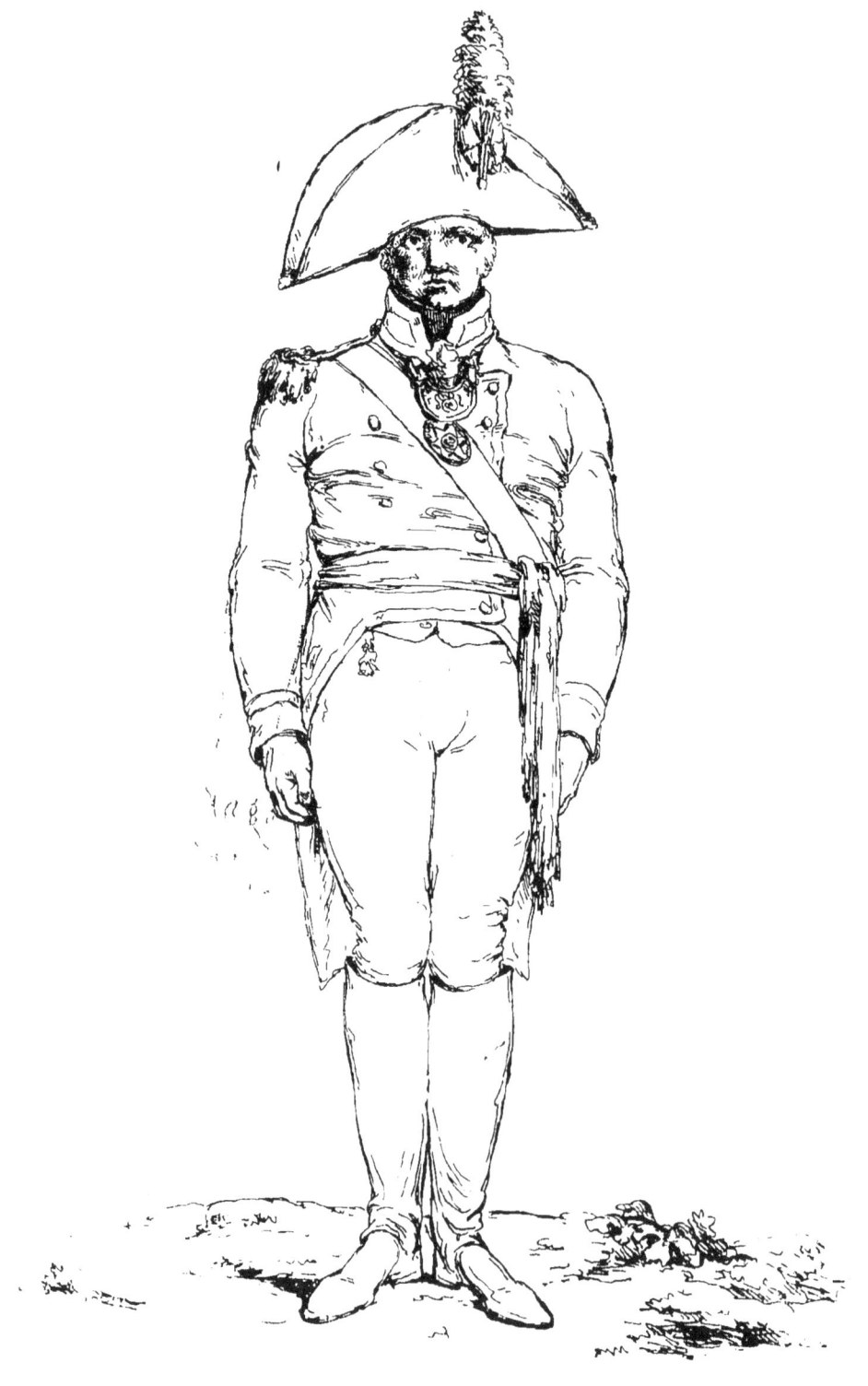

MILITARY INSTRUCTIONS:

INCLUDING

EACH PARTICULAR MOTION

OF THE

MANUAL AND PLATOON EXERCISES;

ELUCIDATED

WITH VERY MINUTE DRAWINGS

BY

Mr R. K. PORTER;

AND DEDICATED WITH PERMISSION TO

LIEUTENANT GENERAL

THE EARL OF HARRINGTON.

BY

DAVID ROBERTS,

LIEUTENANT AND ACTING ADJUTANT OF THE
FIRST REGIMENT OF LIFE GUARDS.

LONDON:

PRINTED FOR T. EGERTON, AT THE MILITARY LIBRARY, NEAR WHITEHALL.

MDCCXCVIII.

TO

LIEUTENANT GENERAL

THE

EARL OF HARRINGTON.

MY LORD,

IN being allowed the honour of dedicating this Work to your Lordſhip, I feel deeply ſenſible of this truth; that it could not be uſhered into the world, under a ſanction more flattering, or more likely to enſure the approbation of the Public.

I have the honour to ſubſcribe myſelf,

My Lord,

Your Lordſhip's

Moſt obedient

And devoted Servant,

DAVID ROBERTS.

PREFACE.

IN prefenting this work to the Public, I muft declare its utility; though I claim no further merit, than the pains which I have taken to pourtray in an accurate and fimple manner, the various motions ufed with the firelock, in the manual and platoon exercifes.

I have been careful moft clofely to conform to the precepts, as *defcribed in the Regulation publifhed by Authority, the 20th of April,* 1792.

I have alfo added fome extra motions, which, though not found in the manual, are of confiderable confequence.

In refpect to thofe inftructions which I offer to officers; I have drawn them from the *beft authorities* :—and as uniformity is effential to every branch of military duty, the pofitions which I have defigned for their rank, will be found as fimple and eafy, as they are true.

With pleafure, I avow myfelf much indebted to my friend Mr. R. K. Porter. He fortunately unites the powers of an artift, to his critical knowledge in military tactics; and has brought forward every exertion on his part, to render the drawings and etchings of this work, worthy the eye of a Martial Public.

INSTRUCTIONS

FOR

PREPARING RECRUITS

FOR THE

Manual Exercise and Ranks.

WHEN a recruit joins the regiment, he will be inſtructed as follows.

The firſt motion—is placing his right foot behind the left, two inches—his left knee bent—and his right thumb cloſed in his left hand.

On the word *Attention*—he will bring up his right foot even with the left, at the ſame time ſtraighten his left knee, forcing it well back, and let his hands fall to each ſide with the thumb a little turned out, and the fingers rather bent inwards, ſo as not to appear ſtiff, forcing back the points of his ſhoulders and neck, raiſing his cheſt well up, and forward, ſo as to throw the weight of his body upon the balls of his feet, in order to obtain a firm poſition, which cannot be the caſe if the weight of the body is leaning backwards upon the heels.

B

For

For the firſt two or three days he muſt then be taught his facings, to the right, and right about ; left and left about.

To Stand at eaſe—with two motions.

The firſt motion—draw the right foot a little behind the left, at the ſame time, making his hands meet acroſs his body, ſtriking one with the other a ſmart pat with the palm; the hands at this time on a line with the elbows—elbows cloſe to the ſides.

The ſecond motion.—Bend the left knee, at the ſame time drop the hands, cloſed as they are, to the waiſtband of the breeches.

The recruit will be then taught to *Salute.*

At one motion—he will raiſe his right hand with an eaſy and graceful motion, to bring the right thumb the height of the right temple, and the fingers extended, in an horizontal line, along the bottom of the hat or cap, the elbow raiſed higher than the ſhoulder, the body quite erect, the head well raiſed, and eyes looking to the front.

N. B. Very particular attention is required from non-commiſſioned officers and privates, to adhere ſtrictly to the foregoing inſtruction whenever they addreſs an officer, or have to *paſs him,* or when an officer *paſſes them.** This is the duty of every non-commiſſioned and private of every regiment, to *all* officers.

---

* Soldiers, alſo with arms, on paſſing an officer or paſſed by any officer, will immediately carry arms until the officer is paſſed, this may be done whilſt in motion.

Facings.

Facings.

Right, Face.	AT the word *Face*, turn the body upon the left heel to the right;—obferve, not to fink or bend the knee, but keep the body erect and fteady.
Right about, Face.	At the word *Face*, drop the right foot back three inches, the ball of the foot oppofite to the left heel; then, with a ftiff knee, turn the body well round to the rear by the right, on the heels : Next motion—bring your right foot back to its proper place.
Left, Face.	As in *Right Face*, only turning on the right heel.
Left about, Face.	Advance the right foot, and bring the heel up to the ball of the left foot, turn round on both heels, knees ftraight, to the rear by the left : Next motion—bring up the right foot to its proper pofition.

HAVING been perfected in the preceding pofitions, the recruit will be taught to *march* in *quick time*—or 120 paces in a minute.

The

The shoulders must be carefully pressed back; the hands hang by the side, but never to appear in front of the thigh, rather behind; the knee that supports the body to be well forced back, which will keep the body steady and preserve the height

Prior to the recruit being put to *slow* time, or 75 paces in the minute, he will be exercised with *dumb-bells* as follows: the dumb-bells being placed one on each side of him, and himself in an erect, steady posture—on the word,

Raise Bells—he will take one in each hand, and by a gentle motion, raise them as high as his arm will suffer him above his head; then gradually sinking them with stretched arm, as much behind him as possible, he will form the circle with them as described in Fig. 1. Plate II. making the circle complete, by causing the backs of his hands to meet behind his body; this will be repeated, according to his strength, five or six times.

Extend Bells.

The bells being raised to the shoulder, they will be forced forwards, keeping the same height, then brought back in the same manner; this will throw the chest forward, and force back the neck and shoulders—this must be frequently repeated

Swing bells.

The top part of the bells to be made meet together in front, the height of the breast; then forced backwards with an extended arm, be made to touch behind: in doing this, the palm of the hands must be uppermost, and the elbows well down . this circle must be repeated 14 or 15 times .—Time, the circle performed, in two seconds.

Ground

Ground Bells.

The recruit will let fall the bells by his fides, and remain fteady and firm.

The recruit will now be taught to march in *ordinary time*, and it will be well to imprefs on his mind, that the word *march*, always implies *ordinary time* when given feparately.

Ordinary time.

The recruit fliding his hands behind him, gradually forces them back (the palms of the hands next the body) until they meet, and then croffing them, with his right he takes a firm hold of the left, then forcing his arms well downwards, ftraightens them and brings his elbows as near together as poffible, raifing his hands a little off from his back, which draws back the points of his fhoulders and opens his cheft, fee Fig. 2. Plate II. In this pofition, he will advance, bringing his breaft well forward, almoft to cover the advancing foot, the toe muft be well pointed, and turned out, then brought to the ground, flat and firm, which if he keeps his body back, he will not be able to do marching in ordinary time. The recruit muft be particular to keep the knee alfo that fupports the body perfectly ftraight.

EVERY recruit fhould be practifed at the balance-ftep, frequently, before the fire-lock is put into his hand.

Left leg, fwing.

The body being perfectly fteady, the left leg raifed from the ground is prefented to the front, loofening the inftep joint, raifing the foot feveral times the height of the right knee, which being as before defcribed, ftraight, and firmly forced back-wards, the body muft be fteady. By a bend of the left knee, the leg will be carried behind, extended well, and raifed up a little; then once more brought to the front, as in the firft pofition.

As you were.

The foot will be brought to the ground, on a line with the right leg ; the fame procefs will be purfued with the right leg.

THE recruit fhould now be taught to *fhoulder* his firelock, and alfo the two firft motions of the *prefent*, to enable him to practife the following exercife, being placed with fhouldered arms.

Sling Arms—from the poife.

The firelock is raifed with the right hand, over the head, the butt to the right, the muzzle to the left, the fore-finger clofe to the top fwivel ; at a fignal, the firelock muft be preffed down-wards to the fhoulder blade; but very great care muft be taken to preferve it exactly fteady, neither fwerving to the right nor the left. In this pofture the balance-ftep muft be prac-tifed. Plate III.

Raife arms.

Raife the firelock above the head, with both hands.

Poife arms.

Letting go the left hand, bring the firelock down with the right hand to the poife, replacing the left hand.

Shoulder

Shoulder Arms.

Throw the firelock well in to the shoulder, and quit the right hand.

It will also be well for the recruit, to practise the following motion:

To Shoulder smartly with one Hand.

Drop the piece from the shoulder with the left hand, into the loading position; then smartly throw it up to the shoulder, using only the left hand.

MUCH care must be taken to habituate men to perform their different duties with regularity; and to instil into their minds, the very great necessity there is for a soldier being strictly attentive, whilst performing any part of his duty. and the moment he falls into the ranks to take up his dressing, to fix himself firmly in his position, and watchfully wait, for any command his officer may give.

Position of the Soldier under Arms.

THE equal squareness of the shoulders, and body, to the front, is the first and grand principle of the position of the soldier:—the heels must be in a line, and closed; the knees straight without stiffness; the toes turned out, so that the feet may form

an

an angle of about 60 degrees ; the arms hang near the body, but not ftiff; the flat of the hand and little finger touching the thigh, and the thumbs as far back as the feams of the breeches ; the elbows and fhoulders are to be kept back ; the belly rather drawn in, and the breaft advanced, but without conftraint ; the body to be upright, but inclining rather forwards, fo that the weight of it may bear chiefly on the balls of the feet ; the head to be erect, and neither turned to the right, nor to the left ; the eyes alone will be glanced to the right.

Under arms, the firelock is to be placed in his left hand, againft the fhoulder ; his wrift to be a little turned out ; the thumb alone to appear in front; the four fingers to be under the butt, and the left elbow to be rather bent inwards, fo as not to be feparated from the body, or to be more backward or forward than the right one ; the firelock muft reft full on the hand, not on the end of the fingers ; and be carried in fuch manner as not to raife, advance, or keep back one fhoulder more than the other ; the butt muft therefore be forward, and as low as can be permitted without conftraint; the fore part a very little before the front of the thigh ; and the hind part of it preffed by the wrift againft the thigh. It muft be kept fteady, and firm, before the hollow of the fhoulder ; fhould it be drawn back, or carried too high, the one fhoulder would be advanced, the other kept back, and the upper part of the body would be diftorted, and not fquare with refpect to the limbs.

Manual

Manual Exercife.

1ft
Order Arms,
(3 motions.)

BRING the firelock to the trail in two   Plate V
motions as ufual, feizing it at the firft, at the
lower loop, juft above the fwell   At the   Fig 1.
fecond, bring it down to the right fide, the
butt within two inches of the ground:—   Fig 2.
At the third, drop the butt on the ground,
placing the muzzle againft the hollow of
the right fhoulder, and the hand flat upon
the fling.   Fig 3

2d
Fix Bayonets.

At the word *Fix*, place the thumb of   Plate VI.
the right hand, as quick as poffible, behind the barrel, taking a gripe of the firelock.—as foon as the word of command is
fully out, pufh the firelock a little forward,
at the fame time drawing out the bayonet
with the left hand, and fixing it with the
utmoft celerity. The inftant this is done,   Fig 1
return, as quick as poffible, to the *Order*,   Fig 2
as above defcribed, and ftand perfectly
fteady. The bayonet muft be feized back-
handed, and well forced down, when in
the act of being drawn out.

C

Shoulder

Plate IV

3d
Shoulder Arms.

As soon as the word *Shoulder* is given, take a gripe of the firelock with the right hand, as in fixing bayonets; and at the laſt word, *Arms*, the firelock muſt be thrown with the right hand, in one motion, and with as little appearance of effort as poſſible, into its proper poſition on the left ſhoulder;—the hand croſſes the body in ſo doing, but muſt inſtantly be withdrawn.

Plate VI
Fig 3

Fig 4

4th
Preſent Arms,
(3 motions.)

Plate VII

1ſt. Seize the firelock with the right hand, under the guard, turning the lock to the front, but without moving it from the ſhoulder.

2d. Raiſe the firelock to the *Poiſe* with the right hand, ſtriking it ſmartly with the left, the fingers extended along the ſling, the wriſt upon the guard, and the point of the left thumb of equal height with the eyes

3d. Bring down the firelock with a quick motion, as low as the right hand will admit without conſtraint, turning the ſling to the front, drawing back the right foot at the ſame inſtant, ſo that the hollow of it may touch the left heel. The firelock in this poſition is to be totally ſupported in the left hand; the butt perpendicular down the center of the left thigh; the body to reſt entirely on the left foot; both knees to be ſtraight.

5th

5th

Shoulder Arms,

(2 motions.)

{ 1ft. By a turn of the right wrift, bring the *Plate IV*
firelock to its proper pofition on the fhoulder,
the left hand grafping the butt. 2d. Quit the
right hand, ·bringing it brifkly down to its *Plate VIII.*
Fig 1.
place by the fide.

6th

Charge Bayonets,

(2 motions.)

{ 1ft. At one motion throw the firelock from *Plate VIII.*
the fhoulder acrofs the body, to the diagonal
pofition in Fig. I. Plate VIII. which is known
in many regiments by the name of *Port Arms* *Fig 1*
or *Prepare to Charge,* in which the lock
is to be turned to the front, and at the height
of the breaft; the muzzle flanting upwards, fo
that the barrel may crofs oppofite the point of
the left fhoulder, with the butt proportionally
depreffed; the right hand grafps the fmall of
the butt, and the left holds the piece at the
fwell, clofe to the lower pipe, the thumbs of
both hands pointing towards the muzzle.

2d. Make a half face to the right, and bring
down the firelock to nearly a horizontal pofiti- *Fig 2*
on, with the muzzle inclining a little upwards,
and the right wrift refting againft the hip.

N. B. The firft motion of the *Charge* is the pofition which
the foldier will, either from the fhoulder, or after firing, take,
in order to advance on an enemy, whom it is intended to attack
with fixed bayonets; and the word of command for that purpofe

C 2

is " *Prepare to Charge.*" The second position of the charge is that which the front rank takes, when arrived at a few yards distance only, from the body to be attacked. The first motion of the *charge* is also that which sentries are to take, when challenging any persons who approach their post.

7th
Shoulder arms.
(2 motions.)

1st—Face to the front, and throw up the piece into its position on the shoulder by a turn of the right wrist, instantly grasping the butt, as before described, with the left hand.

2d—Quit the firelock briskly with the right hand, bringing it to its proper place by the side.

Plate IX

Fig 1

Support Arms.

Fig 2

The men must be taught likewise to *support arms* at *three* motions, throwing the first and second nearly into one : At the first motion, they seize the small of the butt, under the lock, with the right hand, bringing the butt in front of the groin, and keeping the lock somewhat turned out ; at the second, they bring the left arm under the cock ; at the third, they quit the right hand. In *carrying arms* from the *support*, the motions are exactly reversed.

In marching any distance, or in standing at ease when *supported*, the men are allowed to bring their right hands across the body,

body, to the fmall of the butt, which latter muft, in that cafe, be thrown ftill more forward; the fingers of the left hand being uppermoft, muft be placed between the body and the right elbow, Plate 13. The right hands are to be inftantly removed when the divifion *halts*, or is ordered to *drefs by the right*. When ftanding at eafe with fupported arms, the left knee is to be bent, and right foot drawn back fix inches. At the word, *Attention*, the right hand removed, the butt thrown back, and the right leg brought up; left knee ftraightened.

Unfix Bayonets. {

At the word *Unfix*, flip the right thumb in rear of the barrel.— On the word *Bayonets*, with the right hand pufh the firelock forward, fo as to fee the muzzle without inclining the head; with the left hand, feize the focket of the bayonet with the thumb and fore finger, difengage the bayonet from the firelock, and holding it between the finger and thumb, (as in Plate IX No. 3) let it fall by forming a circle, (as in Fig 4,) it will by that motion meet the palm of the hand, and being grafped by the other fingers, the point will be in a pofitive direction to the mouth of the bayonet fcabbard, and cafily returned, the firelock thrown back to the right fhoulder, and the left hand well down to the left fide.*

Plate IX.

Fig 3

Fig 4

*In the above method of returning the bayonet, the men may be allowed to feize the belt, with the right finger and thumb, below the breaft-plate, in order to fteady it

Secure

(14)

Plate X
Fig. 1.

Secure Arms.

Fig 2

Bring the right hand fmartly acrofs the body, fo as to grafp the firelock below the lock; then with the left hand catch the fire-lock near the fwell, and at the fame time fink the muzzle till the butt becomes even with the back of the fhoulder; the lock will be received, and covered by the infide of the bend of the arm.

Shoulder Arms

The muzzle will be flung up to the fhoul-der, the right hand will grafp the fmall of the ftock as in the firft motion (in order to fteady it); the left hand will feize the fire-lock at the butt, and the right hand be then withdrawn.

Plate X.

Fig 4

Ground Arms.

From the *Order*, turn the firelock with the right hand, fo much to the right as to have the lock quite behind; and at the fame time difengage the right foot, and make a half face to the right, fo that the flat of the butt fhall be oppofite the ball of the great toe.—Then advance the left foot, and extend the firelock eafily on the ground, which is done by finking on your right knee, which fhould cover the lock, the left leg perpendicular, and the left hand refting on the calf. The

firelock

firelock is to be laid on the ground, exactly straight from the right foot; the body as nearly erect as possible, the head up, and the eyes to the flugel man. With a spring, which will be much aided by the left hand having grasped the calf of the left leg, the body is to be raised to the perpendicular position, hands down; and the right foot disengaging from the butt of the firelock resumes its proper position, as the body returns with a half face to the front.

Take up Arms. Half face to the right—the right foot placed behind the butt, the body is once more sunk as in Plate XI. the right hand seizing the piece at the swell; the left, the calf of the left leg —the body is again raised to the erect position, excepting that the right hand, during the time the body is rising, slips gradually to the muzzle of the firelock, as in Fig. 3. Disengage the right foot, and bring the body square to the front, the right hand grasping the muzzle as in Fig. 4

Plate XI

Plate X
Fig. 3

Fig. 4

Lase Arms. The right hand is smartly dropped to its length, as in ordered arms

Plate V
Fig. 3

Trail

Trail Arms.	{ The firelock is lifted from the *order*, two inches from the ground, *exactly* in the same position.

Recover from Order or Trail.	{ Fling the firelock with the right hand up to the left shoulder, catching it with the left hand about fix inches above the guard, and with the right close below the guard; the piece perpendicular, and the fling to the front; elbows close as possible to the body.

Plate XXI
Fig 1

————————————

Regular System of Inspection of all Guards, Parties, &c.

EACH foldier falls in with his arms shouldered, touching his right hand man eafy, and dreffing well to the right; when the right hand man finds his left perfectly steady, he orders his arms, and stands at cafe, and so on from right to left of the rank, fingly, man by man, taking care to keep the left foot firm on the ground, in order to remain in drefs. When the *Inspecting Officer* gives the word *Attention*, they will spring smartly up; then the line will be perfectly dreffed, and every man at his proper diftance. The above inftructions to be strictly attended to at all parades.

Words

Words of Command, for inspecting Arms.
{
Fix Bayonets.   Plate VI.

Shoulder Arms.   Plate IV

Open Pans.   Plate XII Fig 1

Port Arms.   Plate VIII Fig 1.

Shoulder Arms.   Plate IV

Shut Pans.   Plate XII. Fig 2.

Order Arms.   Plate V.

Draw Ramrods.   Plate XII. Fig. 3

Return Ramrods.   Plate XII Fig. 4

Order Arms.   Plate V Fig 2

Ease Arms.   Plate V Fig 3

Return Bayonet.   Plate IX Fig 3 and 4

Stand at ease.
}

Fix Bayonets.   {   As in the Manual Exercise.

Shoulder Arms.   {   As in the Manual Exercise.

Open Pans.   { Plate XII. No. 1 —Bring the right hand smart across the body, the thumb under the steel, the fingers over it; by a signal from the corporal advanced, the pan is thrown open . The third motion—the right hand brought smart down by the side.

D

Port

| Plate VIII Fig 1. | Port Arms. | Is to be as the first motion of *Charge Bayonet*, in the Manual Exercise; the inspecting officer will then examine, very minutely, the lock, brasses, and all parts of the firelock below the top swivel. |

| Plate IV | *Shoulder Arms.* | As in the Manual Exercise. |

| Plate XII. Fig 2. | *Shut Pans.* | The right hand brought quick across the body, with the fingers extended above the steel; at the signal, a smart pressure of the hand will shut the pan: the next signal, the right hand is brought quick down to the side. |

| Plate V. | *Order Arms.* | As in the Manual Exercise. |

| | *Draw Ramrods.* | 1st—The thumb behind, the same as previous to the shouldering. 2d. Spring the firelock quick out of the right hand into the left, seizing the top of the ramrod with the thumb and fingers of the right hand—and make a half face to the left at the same time. 3d. Bring the ramrod half way out, and seize it back-handed. 4th. Spring it quite out, entering the thick end of the ramrod into the muzzle. 5th. The hand dropt quick to the muzzle. 6th. Seize the |

top

top of the ramrod with the thumb and finger.
7th. Each foldier will let his ramrod fall into
the barrel, man by man, as the infpecting
officer paffes them from right to left.   8th.
Seize the top of the ramrod with the thumb
and finger of the right hand, bringing it half
way out with the back of the hand outwards :
take it quite out, lay the fmall end of the
ramrod on the right fhoulder, the thick
end to reft on the turn of the bayonet. *Plate XII Fig 3*
9th. The infpecting officer will examine the
muzzle of the firelock, the bayonet, and the
top of the ramrod, (in order to fee if the barrel is clean in the infide) from left to right.

Return Ramrods. 10th. When the officer has paffed the left
hand man, he will raife the thick end of his
ramrod upwards, pointing the fmall end in
the loop, fpring it quick down ; feizing the
top with the thumb and finger, bringing it *Fig. 4*
quite home, the muzzle to the hollow of
the left fhoulder, and face fmartly to the
front.

Order

Order Arms. 11th. Bring the fingers of the right hand fmartly round the muzzle, taking a full grafp of it about the fwell. 2d motion—Bring it from the left fide to the right, the left hand to remain ftraight by the fide, the right hand to the muzzle; the butt to the ground, the outfide of the right foot, and within the toe.

Eafe Arms. The right hand to drop fmart upon the fling, with the arm extended, and the back of the hand to the front.

Platoon

Platoon Exercife.

FRONT RANK STANDING.

Prime and Load. {

1ft—Bring the firelock down in one brifk motion to the priming pofition, the thumb of the right hand placed againft the pan cover, or fteel; the fingers clenched, and the elbow a little turned out, fo that the wrift may be clear of the cock. The greateft care fhould be taken to keep the lock well forward, fo that the head need not be at all turned to view it—only a caft of the eye downwards.

2d—Open the pan, by throwing up the fteel, with a ftrong motion of the thumb, forced by the right arm, turning the elbow in, and keeping the firelock fteady in the left hand.

3d —Bring your hand round to the pouch, and draw out the cartridge.

Plate XIV.
Fig. 1

Fig 2

Fig 3.

The reft as above defcribed, excepting, that in the quick loading, all the motions are to be done with as much difpatch as poffible; the foldiers taking their time from the flugel man in front, for *cafting about* and *fhouldering* only.

Priming

Priming Pofition. { In firing three deep, the priming pofition for the front rank is the height of the waiftband of the breeches; for the center rank, about the middle of the ftomach; and for the rear rank, clofe to the breaft :—the firelock in all thefe pofitions, is to be kept perfectly horizontal.

Plate XIX
Fig 1.

1ft

Make Ready. { As ufual, bringing the firelock to the *Recover*, and inftantly cocking.

Plate XX.
Fig. 1

2d

Prefent. { 1ft—Slip the left hand along the fling as far as the fwell of the firelock, and bring the piece down to the *Prefent*, ftepping back about fix inches to the rear with the right foot.

Fig. 2. and 3.

3d

Fire. { After firing drop the firelock brifkly to the *Priming Pofition*.
2d—Half cock.

Plate XIV.
Fig 3

4th

Handle Cartridge. { 1ft—Draw the cartridge from the pouch.
2d—Bring it to the mouth, holding it between the fore finger and thumb, and bite off the top of it.

Fig. 4 and 5.

5th

5th
Prime.

1ſt—Shake ſome powder into the pan.

2d—Shut the pan with the three laſt fingers.

3d—Seize the ſmall of the butt with the above three fingers.

Plate XV.
Fig. 1.

Fig 2.

Fig. 3.

6th
Load.

1ſt—Face to the left on both heels, ſo that the right toe may point directly to the front, and the body be a very little faced to the left, bringing at the ſame time the firelock round to the left ſide without ſinking it. It ſhould, in this momentary poſition, be almoſt perpendicular, (having the muzzle only a ſmall degree brought forward) and as ſoon as it is ſteady there, it muſt inſtantly be forced down within two inches of the ground, the butt nearly oppoſite the left heel, and the firelock itſelf ſomewhat ſloped, and directly to the front; the right hand at the ſame inſtant catches the muzzle, in order to ſteady it.

2d—Shake the powder into the barrel, putting in after it the paper and ball.

3d—Seize the top of the ramrod with the fore finger and thumb.

Fig 4

Plate XVI

Plate XVII.
Fig 1

Fg 2

7th

Fig. 3.

Fig 4.

7th
Draw Ramrods.

> 1ſt—Force the ramrod half out, and ſeize it back-handed exactly in the middle.
>
> 2d—Draw it entirely out, and turning it with the whole hand and arm well extended in front, put it one inch into the barrel.

Fig 5

Fig. 6

8th
Ram down Cartridge.

> 1ſt—Puſh the ramrod down, holding it as before, exactly in the middle, until the hand touches the muzzle.
>
> 2d—Slip the fore finger and thumb to the upper end, without letting the ramrod fall further into the barrel.
>
> 3d—Puſh the cartridge well down to the bottom.
>
> 4th—Strike it two very quick ſtrokes with the ramrod.

Plate XVII.
Fig 3

9th
Return Ramrods.

> 1ſt—Draw the ramrod out, catching it back-handed.
>
> 2d—Draw it entirely out, turning it very briſkly from you, with the arm extended, and put it into the loops, forcing it as quick as poſſible to the bottom; then face to the proper front, the finger and thumb of the right hand holding the ramrod, as in the poſition immediately previous to drawing it, and the butt raiſed two inches from the ground.

Plate XVIII

10th

| 10th Shoulder Arms. | Strike the top of the muzzle fmartly with the right hand, in order to fix the bayonet and ramrod more firmly, and at the fame time throw it nimbly up, at one motion, to the fhoulder. |

N. B. Though the butts are not to come to the ground in cafting about, as accidents might happen from it; yet they are permitted, while loading, to be fo refted, but it muft be done without noife, and in a manner imperceptible in the front.

The Pofition of each Rank in the Firings.

FRONT RANK KNEELING.

| Make Ready. | BRING the firelock brifkly up to the Recover, catching it in the left hand, and without ftopping, fink down with a quick motion upon the right knee, keeping the left foot faft; the butt end of the firelock, at the fame moment, falling upon the ground; then cock, and inftantly feize the cock and fteel together in the right hand, holding the piece firm in the left, about the middle of that part which is between the lock and the fwell of the ftock: |

E

ſtock ; the point of the thumb to be cloſe to the ſwell, and pointing upwards. As the body is ſinking, the right knee is to be thrown back, that the left leg may be right up and down; the right foot a little turned out; the body ſtraight, and the head as much up, as if ſhouldered : the firelock muſt be upright, and the butt about four inches to the right of the inſide of the left foot.

Plate XIX
Fig 1. and 2

Plate XX.

Preſent.

Bring the firelock down firmly to the *Pre-ſent*, by ſliding the left hand, to the full extent of the arm, along the ſling, without letting the motion tell; the right hand at the ſame time ſpringing up the butt, ſo high againſt the right ſhoulder, that the head may not be too much lowered in taking aim; the right cheek cloſe to the butt; the left eye ſhut, and the middle finger of the right hand on the trigger; look along the barrel with the right eye, from the breech pin to the muzzle, and remain ſteady.

Fire.

Pull the trigger ſtrong with the middle finger; and as ſoon as fired, ſpring up nimbly upon the left leg, keeping the body erect, and the left foot faſt ; bringing the right heel to the hollow of the left ; at the ſame inſtant, ftant, drop the firelock to the priming pofition, the height of the waiftband of the breeches; *Half Cock*; *Handle Cartridge*, and go on with the loading motions, as before defcribed.

Plate XX.
Fig 1, 2,
and 3.

·

CENTER RANK.

Make Ready.

SPRING the firelock brifkly to the *Recover*; as foon as the left hand feizes the firelock above the lock, raife the right elbow a little, placing the thumb of that hand upon the cock, with the fingers open on the plate of the lock, and then, as quick as poffible, cock the piece, by dropping the elbow and forcing down the cock with the thumb, ftep at the fame time with the right foot a moderate pace to the right, keeping the left faft; feize the fmall of the butt with the right hand. The piece muft be held in this pofition perpendicular, and oppofite the left fide of the face, the butt clofe to the breaft, but not preffed; the body ftraight, and full to the front, and the head erect.

Plate XXI.
Fig. 1

Prefent.

As in the foregoing explanation for the front rank.

Plate XX.

E 2

Pull

Fire.

Pull the trigger ftrong with the middle finger, and as foon as fired, bring the firelock to the priming pofition, about the height of the ftomach; the reft, as in explanation of *Priming* and *Loading*;—with this difference only, that the left foot is to be drawn up to the right, at the fame time that the firelock is brought down to the priming pofition; and that immediately after the firelock is thrown up to the fhoulder, the men fpring to the left again, and cover their file leaders.

Plate XX.

REAR RANK.

Make Ready.

RECOVER and cock, as before directed for the center rank; and as the firelock is brought to the *Recover*, ftep brifkly to the the right a full pace, at the fame time placing the left heel about fix inches before the point of the right foot. The body to be kept ftraight, and as fquare to the front as poffible.

Plate XXI
Fig 2

Prefent.

As in directions for the center rank; only leaning well on the left foot.

Fire.

Fire. { As in directions for the center rank ;—remembering only the difference of the priming position for this rank, as before defcribed; after firing and fhouldering, the men ftep as the center rank does.

Plate XX.

N. B. In firing with the front rank *ftanding*; that rank makes ready, &c. as fpecified in the article relative to the *Platoon Exercife.*

Firing by Platoons.

THE officers, inftead of giving the words, *Platoon, Make Ready, Prefent, Fire*; are to pronounce the words fhort, as tor inftance, *'Toon, Ready, 'Pfent, Fire.*

In firing by platoons or divifions, the officers commanding them are to ftep out one pace, on the clofe of the *Preparative*, and face to the left towards their men; they there ftand perfectly fteady till the laft part of the *General,* when they ftep back again into their proper intervals, all at the fame time. After a divifion has fired, the right hand man of it fteps out one pace, in front of the officer, but ftill keeping his own proper front, and gives the time for *cafting about* and *fhouldering*, after which he falls back again into his place in the front rank.

The flugel man of a battalion is alfo to keep his front, in

giving

giving the time of exercife. In firing by grand divifions, the center officer falls back, on the *Preparative,* into the fourth rank, and is replaced by the covering ferjeant.

Pile or File Arms.

THIS is done from the *Order, Front Rank to the Right about, Face* ; at the fame moment the center rank makes a quarter face to the left ; throwing the firelock out of the right hand into the left, and fpringing the butt againft the left heel, with the lock ' outwards. The rear rank brings the right hand to the muzzle of the firelock, and fprings the butt againft his right heel, with the lock to the rear. The files flope their arms, lock their ramrods in each other, and fo form the complete pile.

Stand Clear Arms. { The front rank ftep back one pace ; the center one, and the rear two. If there are only two ranks file, the rear muft *take open order* ; the front to the right about, when they lock arms to the right alternately, viz. two fronts, one rear ; and two rear, and one front.

To

Unfile Arms.

{ To *Stand to Arms*, each man grasps his piece with his left hand; at the word *Arms*, the front rank faces to the right about, and each man throws his firelock from his left hand into his right;—and so is again in order.

Instructions for Serjeants.

THE serjeants carrying halberts, will shoulder their halbert on the right side, in a manner similar to that of shouldering the firelock on the left, letting the point of the staff rest between the two first fingers. They will order in three motions.

1st motion. Seize the halbert with the left hand opposite the point of the right shoulder.

2d motion. Raise the right hand to catch the halbert, about two inches above the left hand, keeping the elbow close to the side.

3d motion.—Sink the halbert to the ground, with the right hand, the left falling to its first position.

When the battalion shoulder, the serjeant will shoulder his halbert, the motion exactly the same as with the firelock, only on the right side,—in two motions.

1st

1st motion—On the word *Shoulder* take a grafp of the halbert with the right hand.

2d motion—Throw the halbert lightly to the right fhoulder, catching it with the right hand.

When the battalion charge, the ferjeants will *Charge Halberts*, in two motions.

Plate XXIV 1st motion, as the firft motion of the *Order*.

2d motion—Raife the right hand till the knuckles reft upon the rear of the right hip, the left hand will bring down the point of the halbert to about the height of the chin.

Serjeants remain at the *Shoulder* during the performance of the other parts of the exercife: there being the fame number of motions for the *Shoulder*, *Order* and *Charge* with the halbert as with the firelock, the fame time will be obferved whilft performing thofe motions.

Instructions for Officers.

THE position of an officer is exactly the same as that de-scribed for the private. Officers must draw their swords on taking their posts in the ranks

Draw Swords. {

I have described the first position in Plate I. Having with the left hand seized the scabbard as near the top as the belt will admit; the sword must be raised perpendicular, so as to meet the right hand. The right hand, at the time the left seizes the scabbard, will be brought, with a quick motion, across the body, so as to clasp the hilt, if not with a full grasp, as near as possible to do it with ease, and the motion graceful

Plate XXII
Fig 1.

The next motion is to draw the sword swiftly out of the scabbard, and bring it to the recover. The right hand will draw the sword, and with a graceful motion raise the hilt in front of the face; the flat of the blade opposite to the nose, and the tip of the thumb on an equal height with the bottom of the chin.

Fig 2.

F

If the ranks are at *Clofe Order*, the officer will *flope his fword*; the right hand will be lowered with the fword, juft fo far on the right fide as to admit of the hand keeping a firm grafp of the hilt; and being brought well fquare to the front, the blade will fall upon the right fhoulder, where it will be held fteady and firm.

Plate XXII.
Fig 3

When the ranks are at open order, the fword will be extended diagonally acrofs the body, from the right fide to the point of the left fhoulder; the right arm being ftraightened perpendicularly down the right fide, the left arm will be bent, fo that the left hand may take the blade of the fword, edgeways, between the fingers and thumb, and be oppofite to the point of the fhoulder.

Fig 4

In the Salute ftanding, the fword is raifed to the front of the face (as in the *recover*) when the general paffes the next officer on the right; then, when the general or field officer has paffed that officer neareft on the right, the right hand of the faluting officer will at firft flowly move, but when near half the half circle is performed, he will fmartly drop the fword, to point about twelve inches in the front of the toe; but as the fword will be brought down to the fide, fo that the guard will touch the feam of the breeches, the point is confequently held in a ftraight line, about three inches on the right of the right foot; the officer will then look to the front, and ftand very fteady. When the general has paffed the faluting officer, he will recover his fword as in Fig 2. Plate XXII. then drop it, as in Fig. 4.

In marching in open ranks, the fword is carried, as in Fig 3.
Plate

Plate XXII. In *faluting*, the officer muft be careful to look direct at the officer *faluted*. He muft by no means begin his falute, till the rear rank of the divifion in his front, are three paces paft the general. The fword will then be recovered, as in Fig. 2. Plate XXII. beginning the firft motion with the right leg, then waiting one ftep, and dropping the fword; with the right leg, exactly to the fame pofition as when faluting ftanding; march three fteps, with the point down; and at the fourth, which will be with the right leg, bring the fword up to the re-cover, wait one ftep, then with the right leg, bring it to Plate XXIII.

N. B. Much attention fhould be given to uniformity in the drefs; and putting the hat properly on the head. And as by conftant attention and practice, the foldier is accuftomed to be extremely firm and fteady in the ranks; it is therefore effentially the duty of an officer, to preferve the fame ftrictnefs; and to let *precept* be fupported by *example*.

Before I conclude, I muft obferve to young officers, the bad effects of confining foldiers by imprifoning them in guard rooms, for fmall and trivial offences. The firft and chief object, when a recruit is to be trained for the ranks, is to teach him regularity and method. His time fhould be fo difpofed and allotted, that every hour in the day fhould be employed: Cleaning himfelf, burnifhing his arms and accoutrements, with the hours ap-

pointed

pointed for drill, and for any other duty which he may be ordered to perform, fuch as *orderly* in barracks, cleaning rooms, cooking for his own meals, &c. may, altogether fo occupy his full time, that little leifure can be left for wafte, in lounging about and drinking. The conftant and regular performance of thefe employments, become habitual, and the foldier goes fucceffively from one duty to another, almoft inftinctively. But if this order and punctuality, is broken through by confinement in his prifon room, the foldier either fleeps all day, or lolls upon benches, regardlefs of his appearance or character; he acquires a habit of indolence, and foon lofes that attention to propriety and regularity, which he had by cuftom obtained; his health fades away before floth and negligence; his mifconduct increafes; and much care and labour muft be exerted, in the attempt to reinftate him as an ufeful and orderly foldier. Hence, I wifh to enforce, that any mode of punifhment is preferable to confinement. For inftance, an increafe of fatigue; the fhame of a turned coat; or any other of thofe modes of difgrace which are daily practifed. In refpect to punifhment, I would always ftrongly recommend that manner, by which the burthen of *duty* fhould fall upon thofe men, whofe conduct has been faulty; by which means, the fatigue of the good men will be lightened, and the award anfwer two purpofes.—punifhing the guilty, and rewarding the meritorious.

THE END.

PLATE II

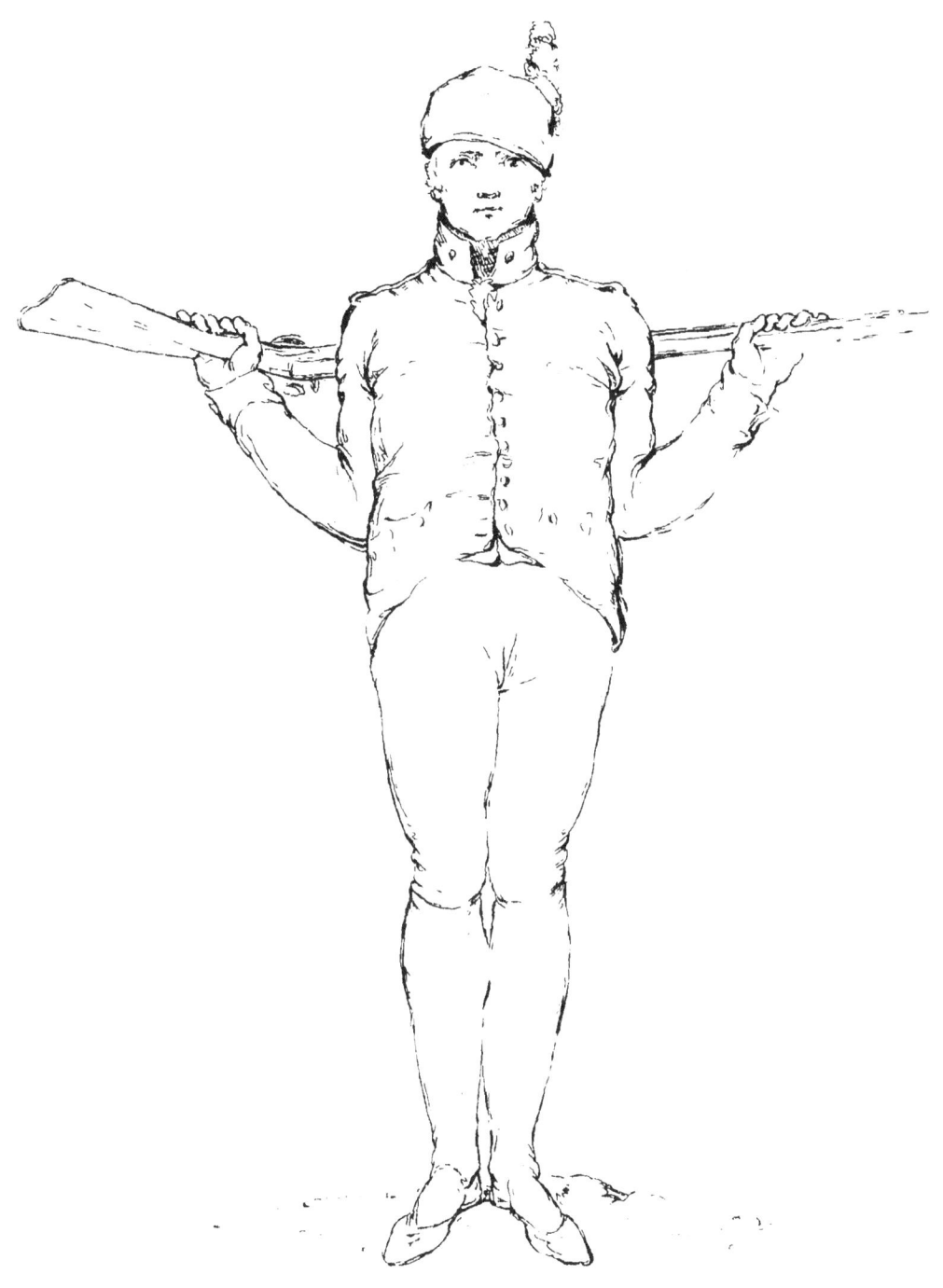

Published as the Act directs Aug.st 10.th 1796 at Egertons Military Library Whitehall

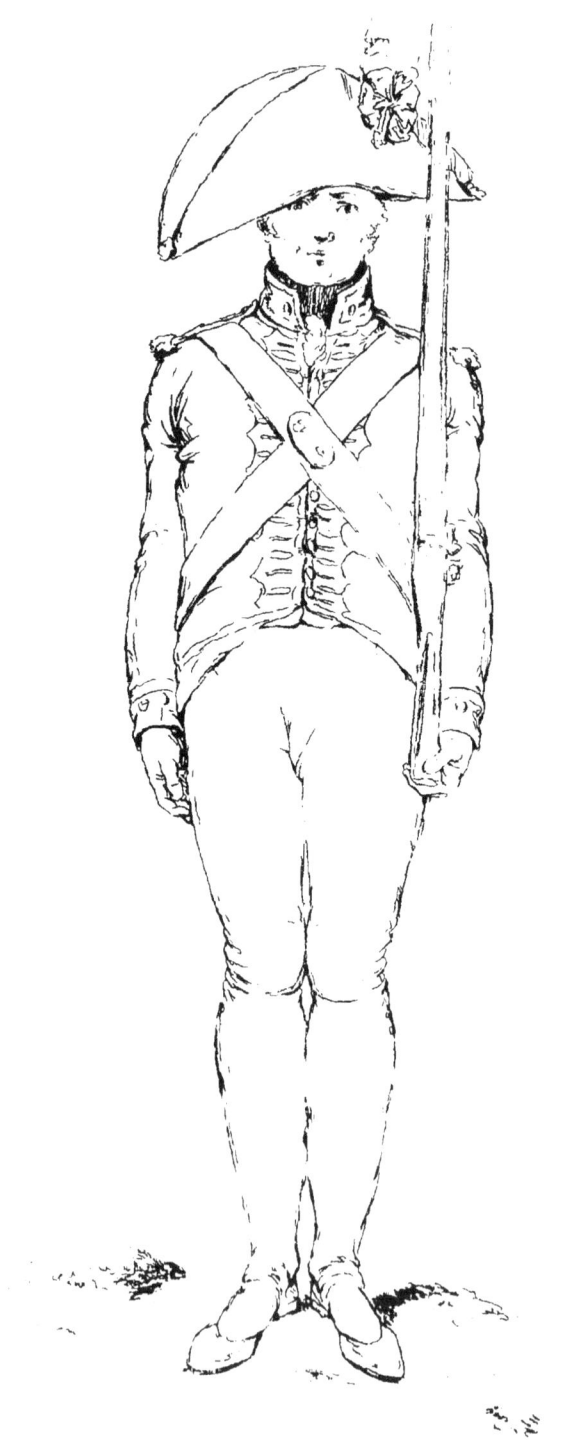

Individuals — — — la — — may 30th 710 at Ipswich Military College Barracks

PLATE V

PLATE VI

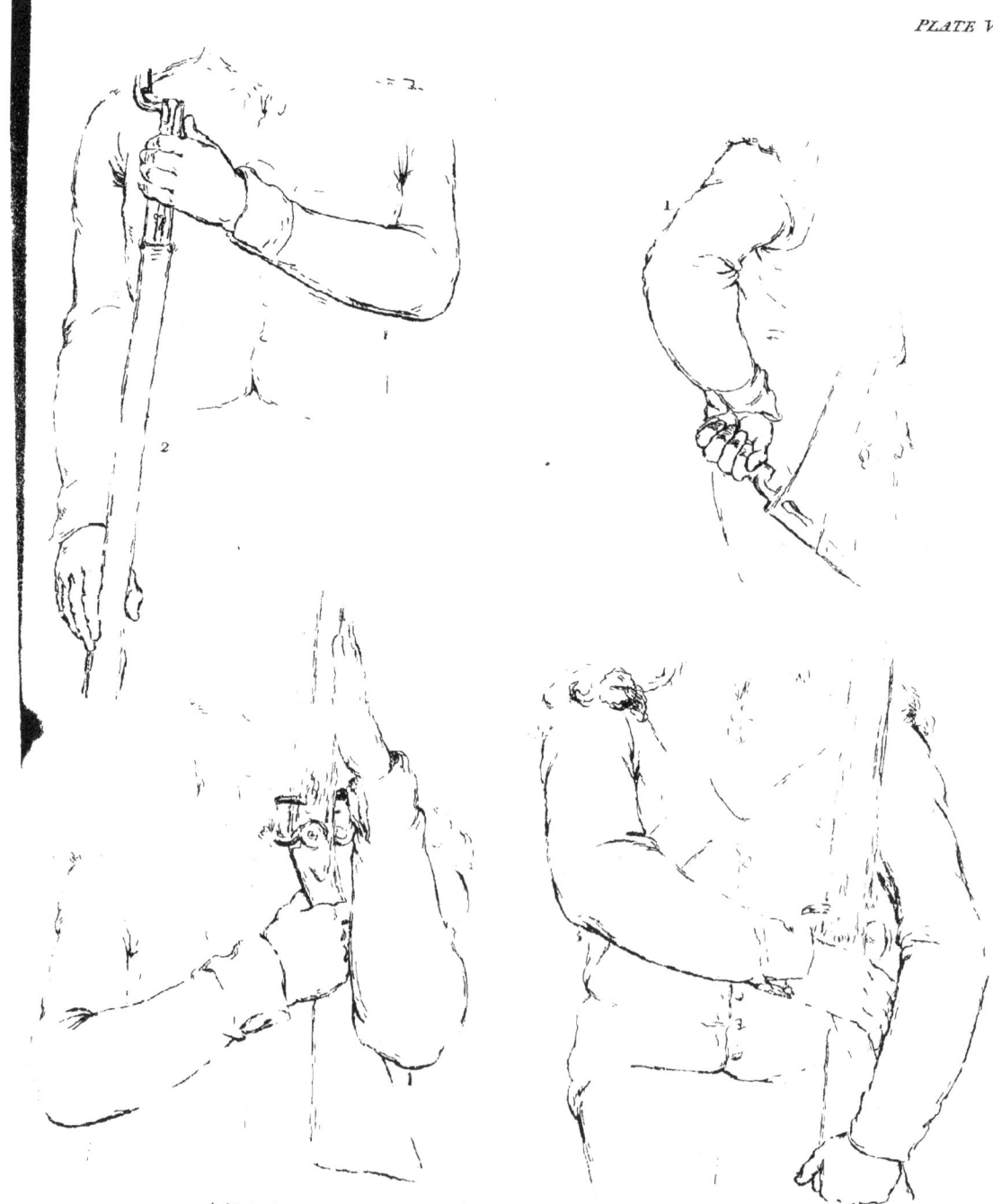

PLATE VII

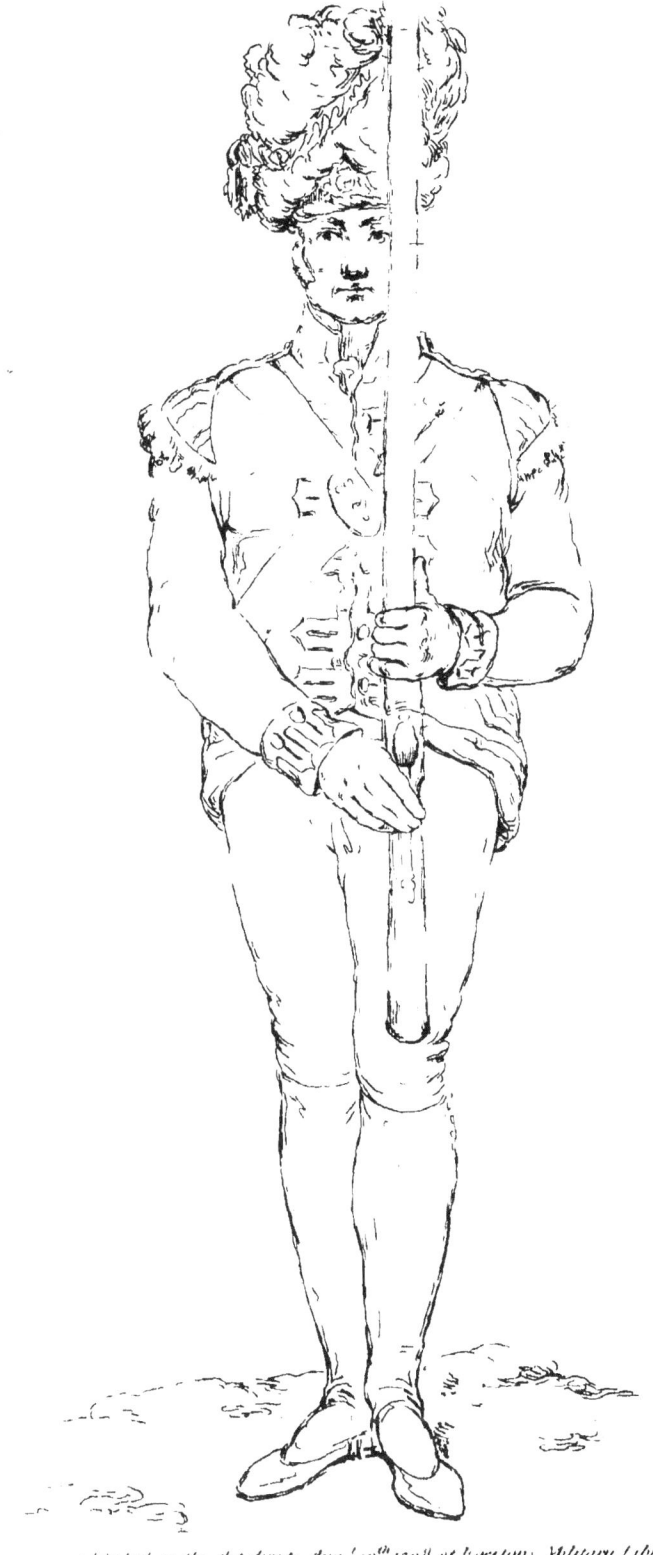

Published as the Act directs Aug.st 30.th 1798 at Egerton's Military Library Whitehall

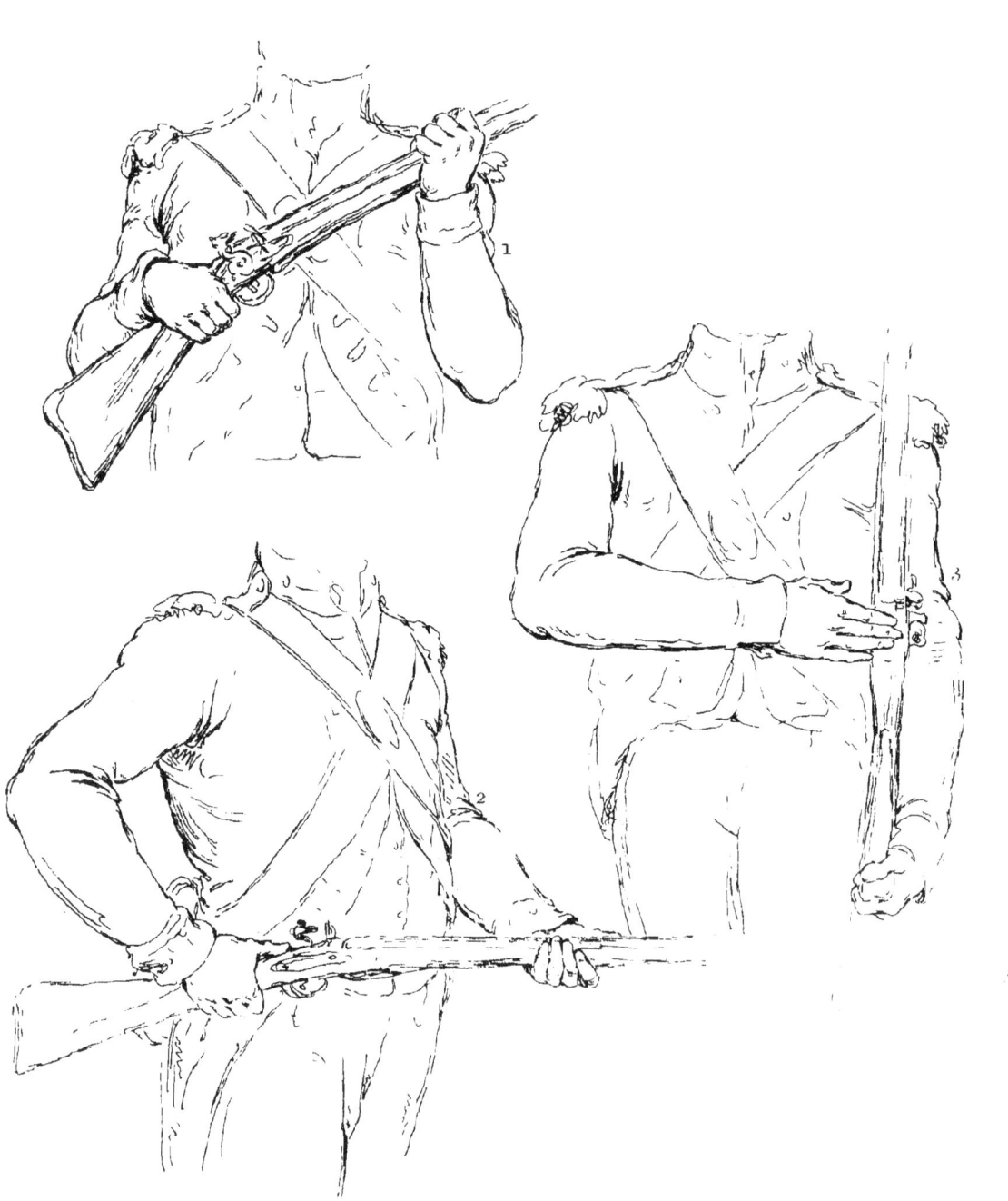

PLATE IX

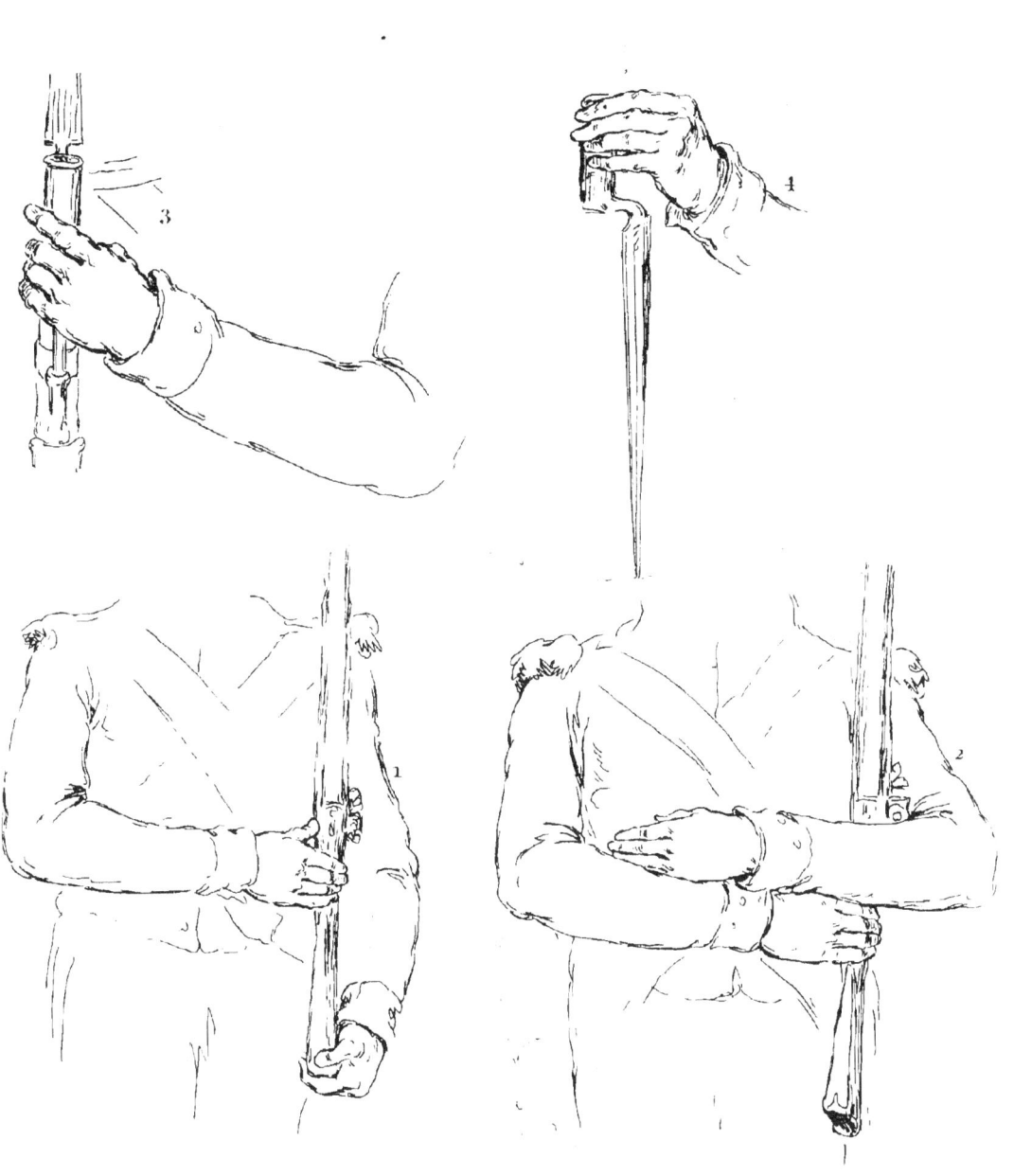

PLATE X.

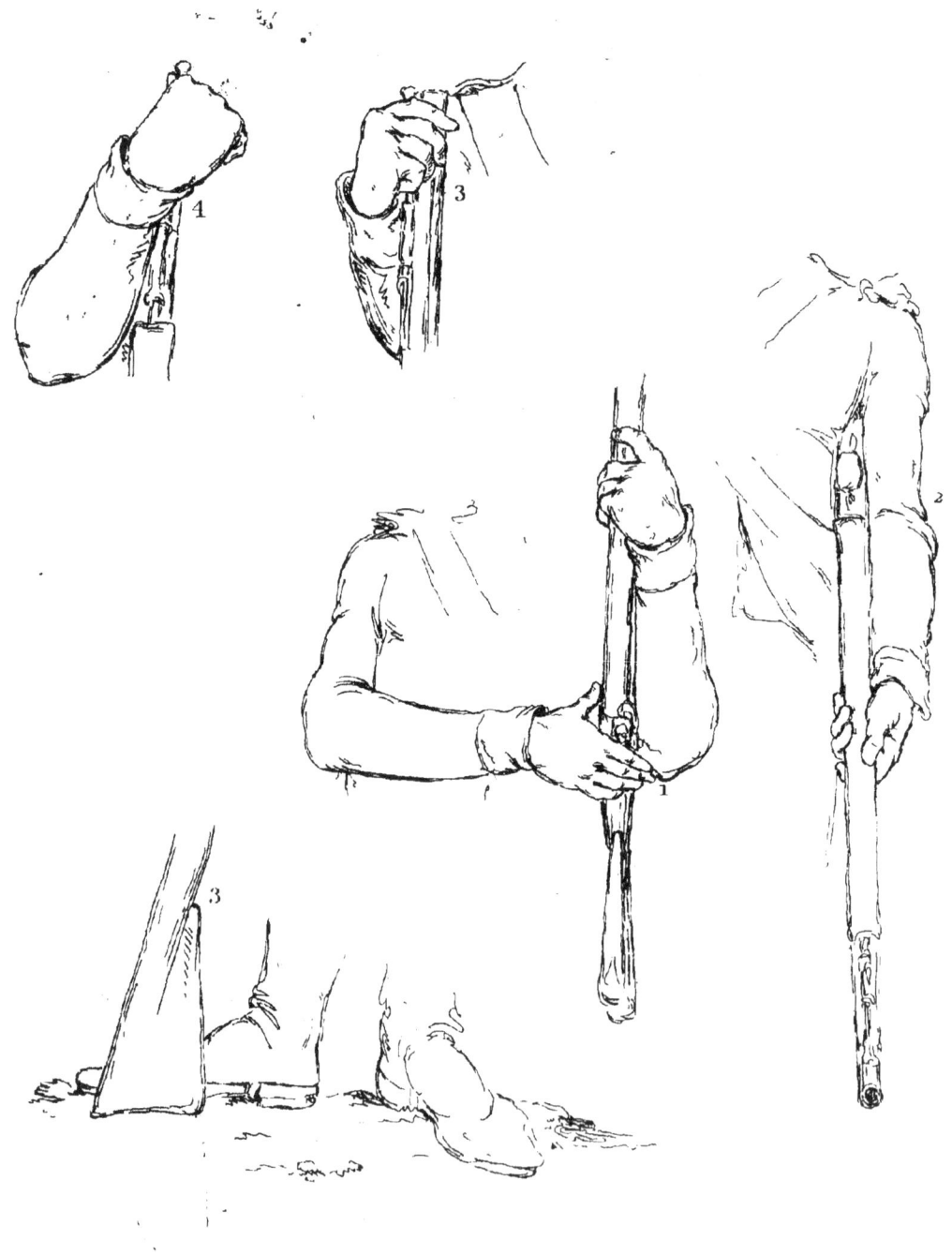

Published as the Act directs Aug.st 10.th 1798 at Egerton's Military Library, Whitehall

PLATE XII

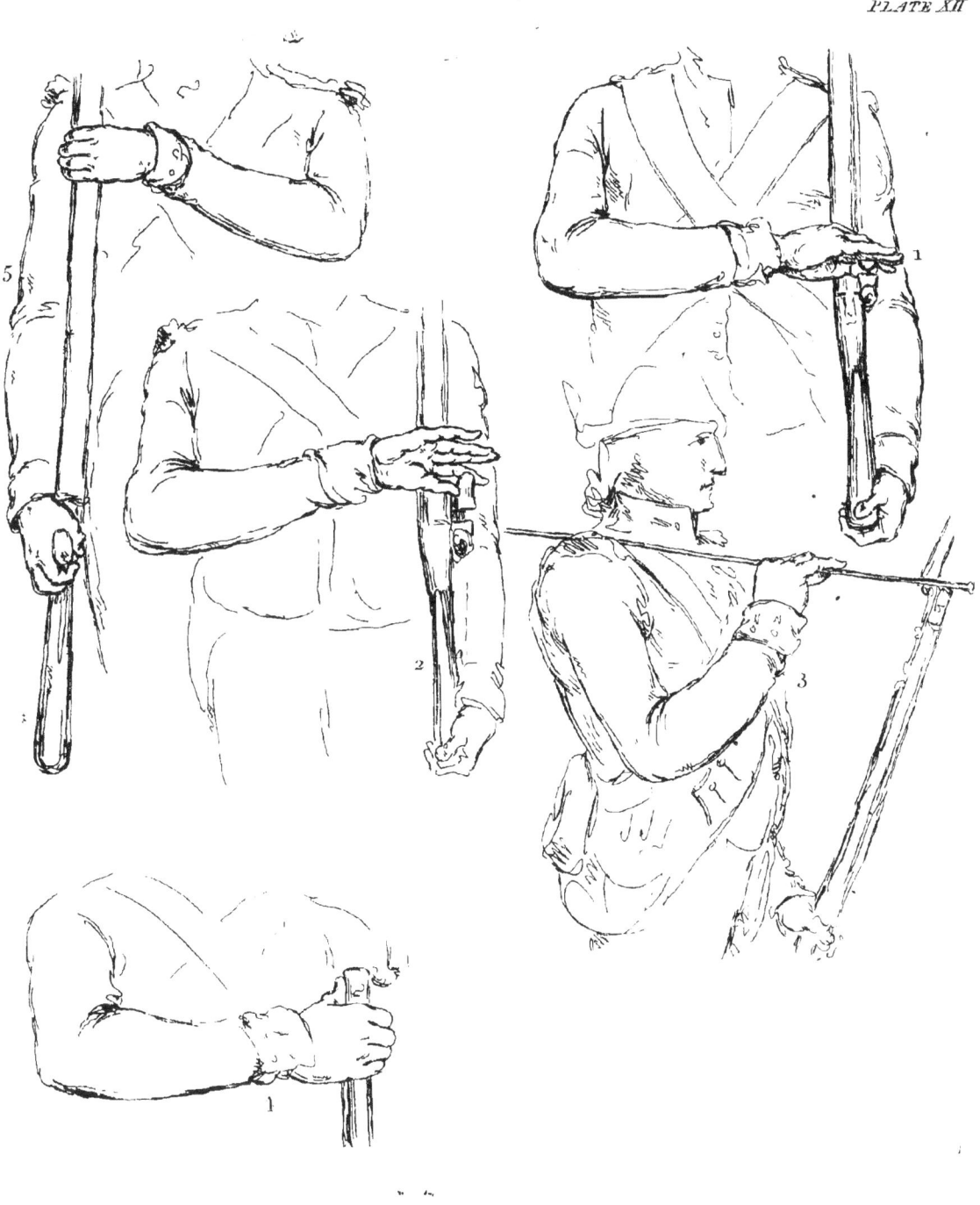

PLATE XIII

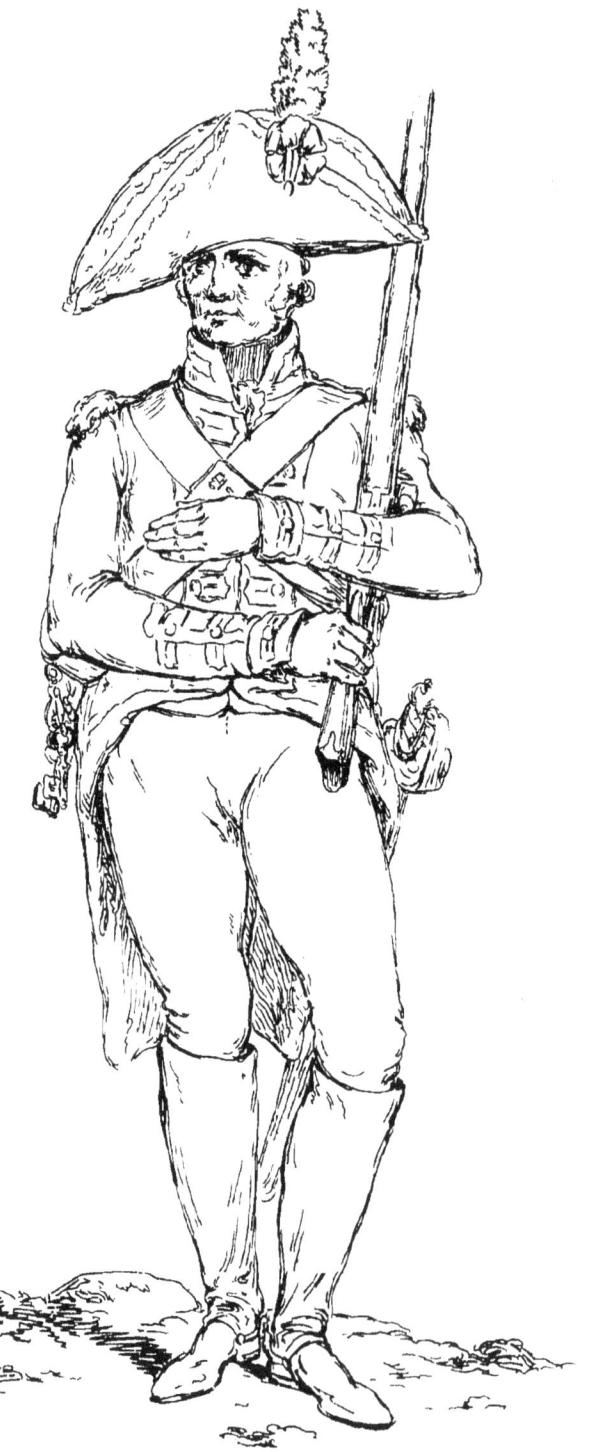

PLATE XIV

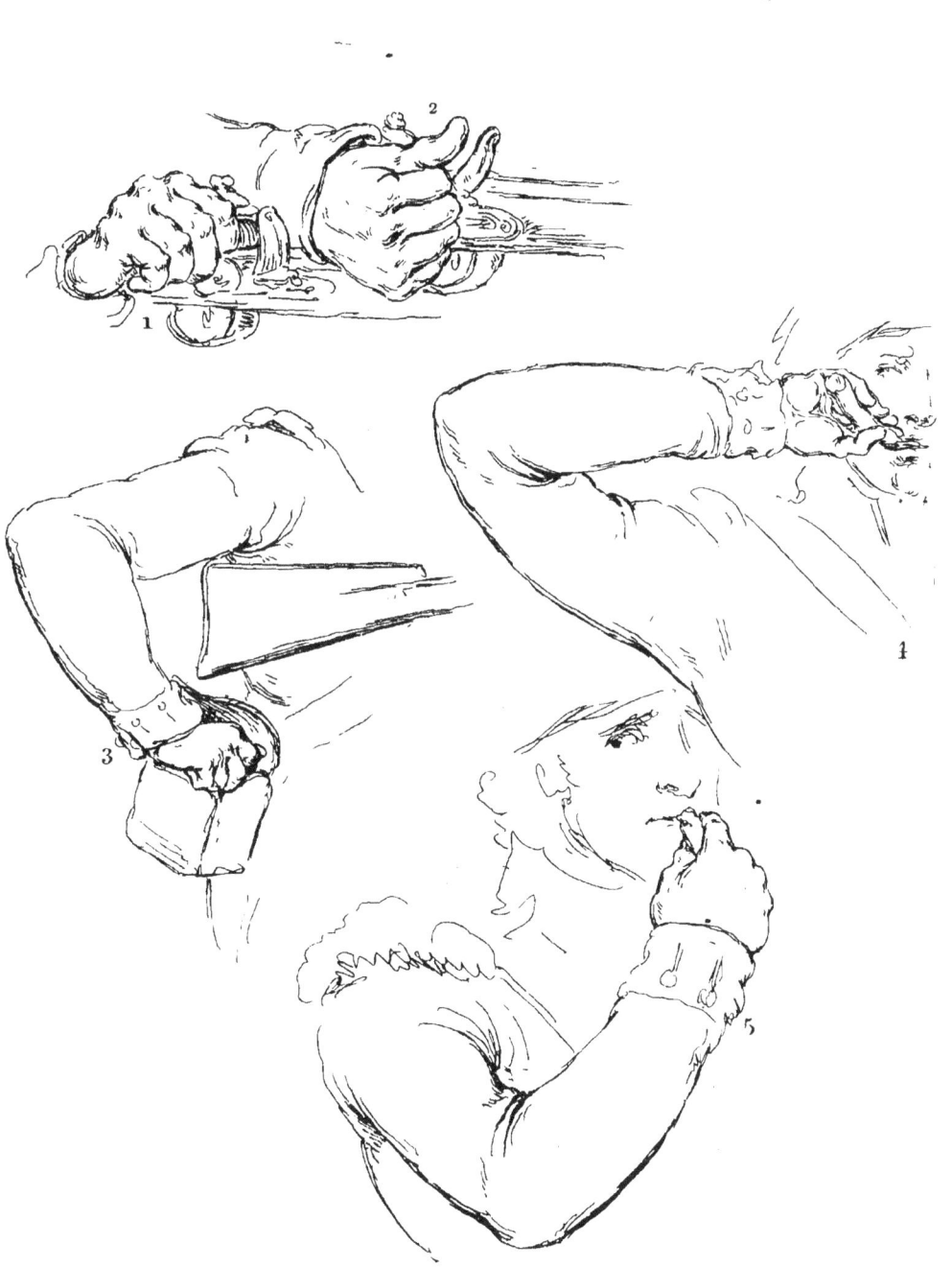

PLATE XV

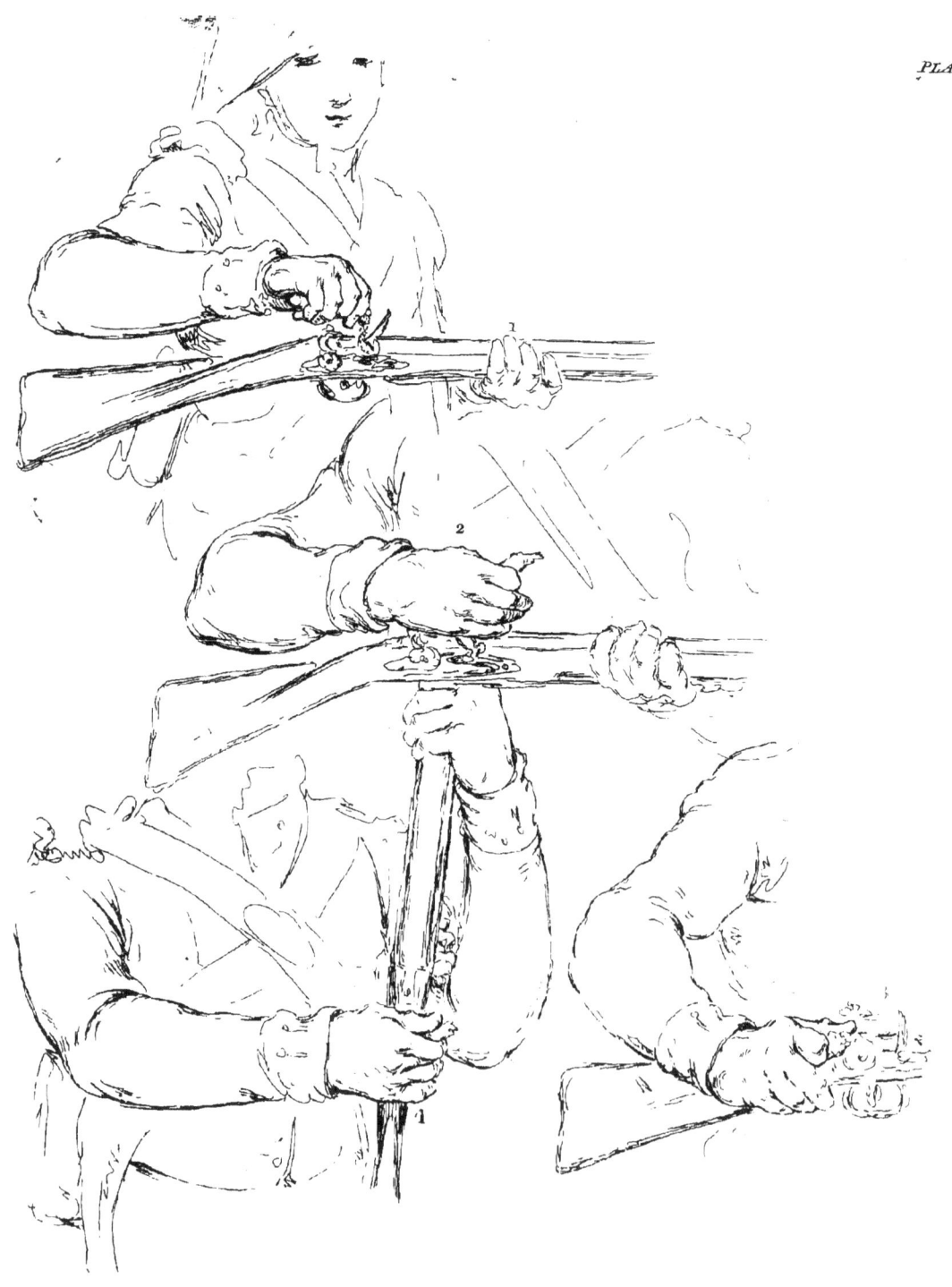

Published as the Act directs Jan.y 1.st 1798, by alexander Melu a, J. I on Hovarall

PLATE XVI.

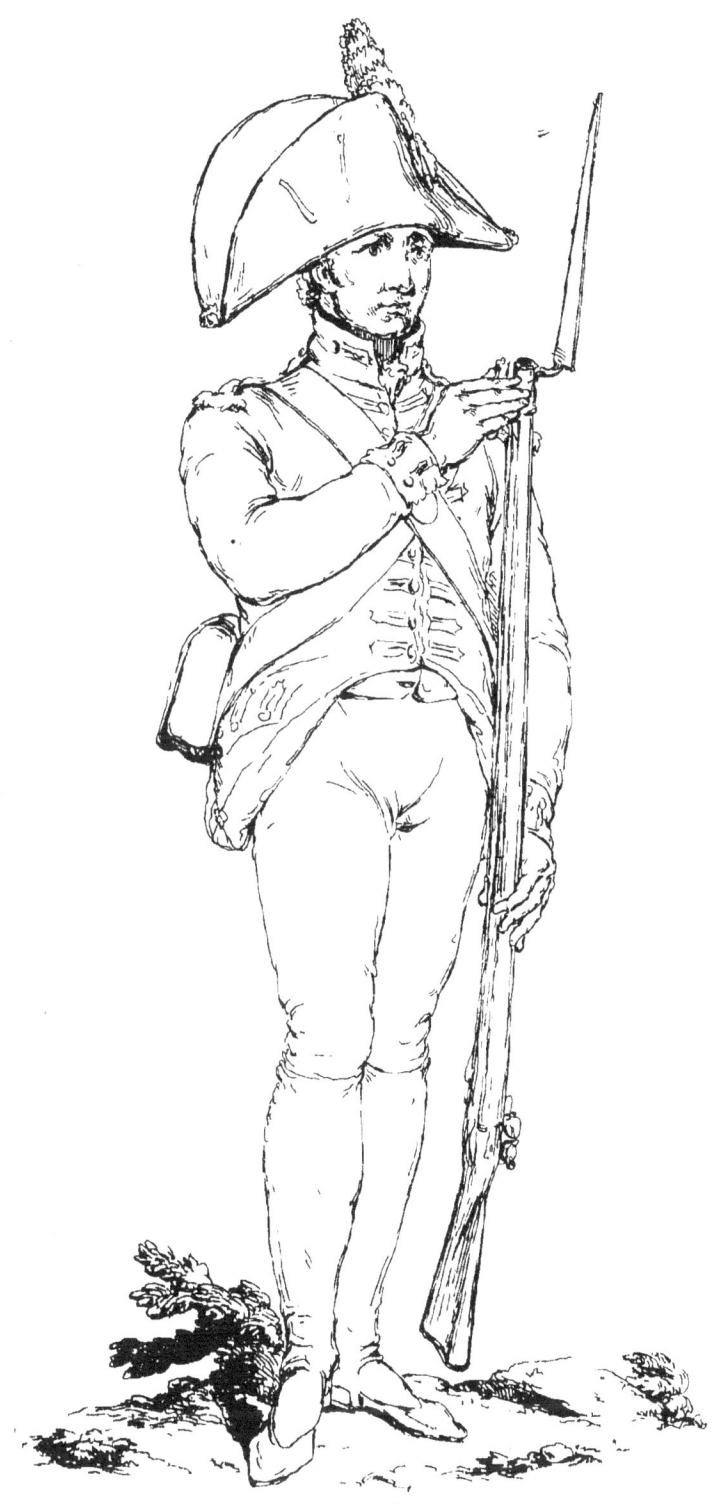

Published as the Act directs Aug.st 30.th 1798, at Egertons Military Library Whitehall

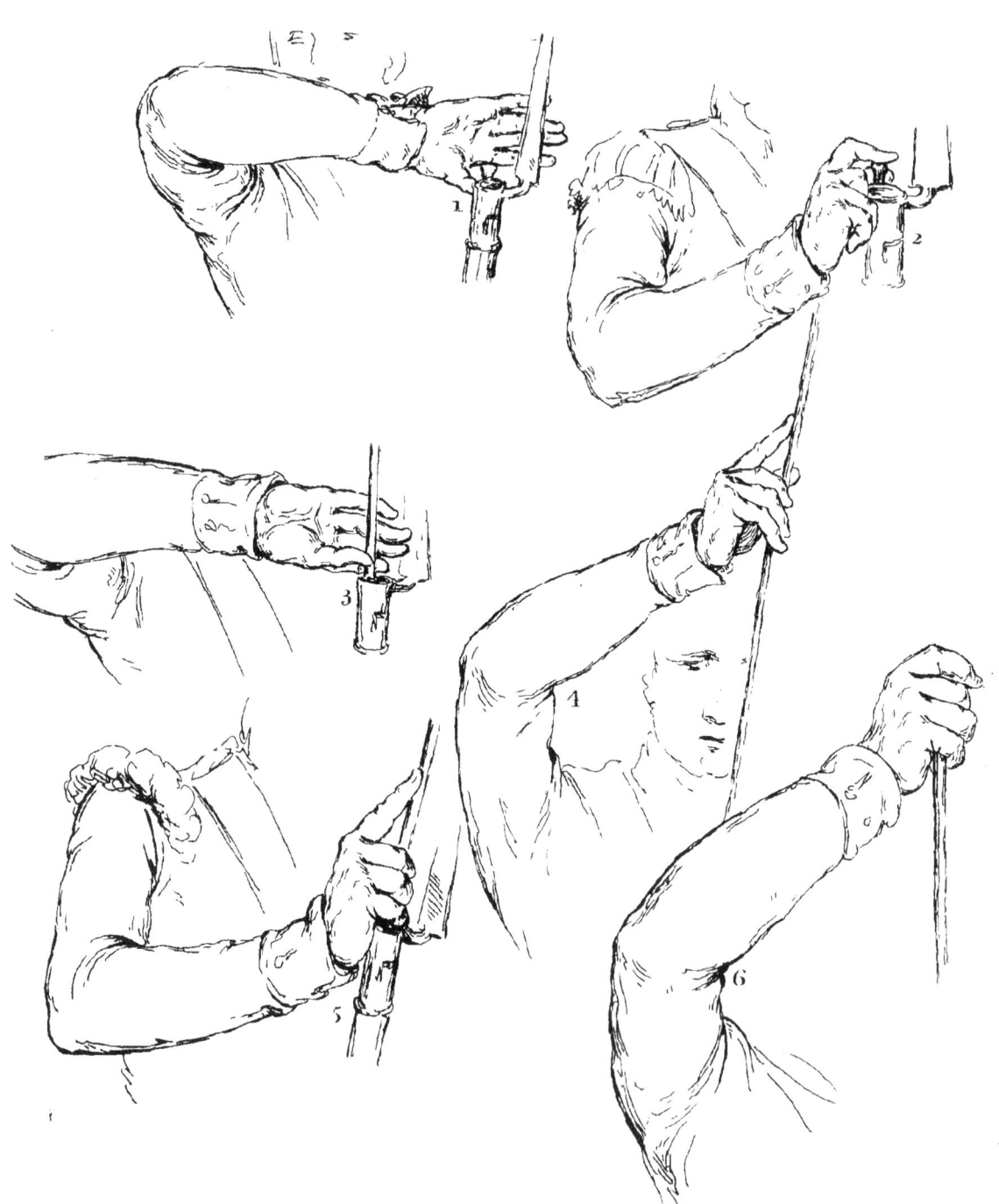

Published as the Act directs, Aug.st 30.th 1790 at Egertons Military Library Whitehall

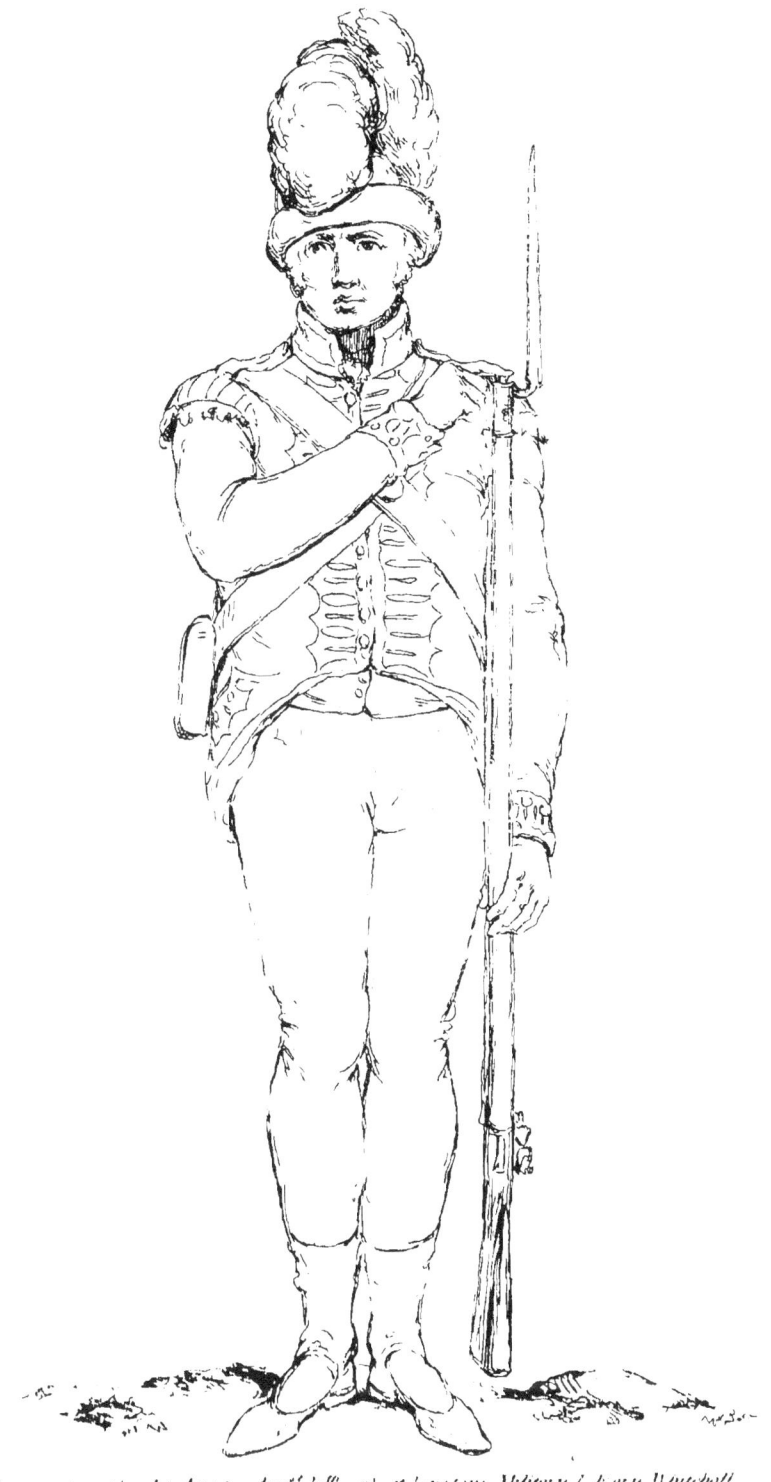

Drawn for the Bedford Augusta Battn of the Loyal London Military Association Whitehall

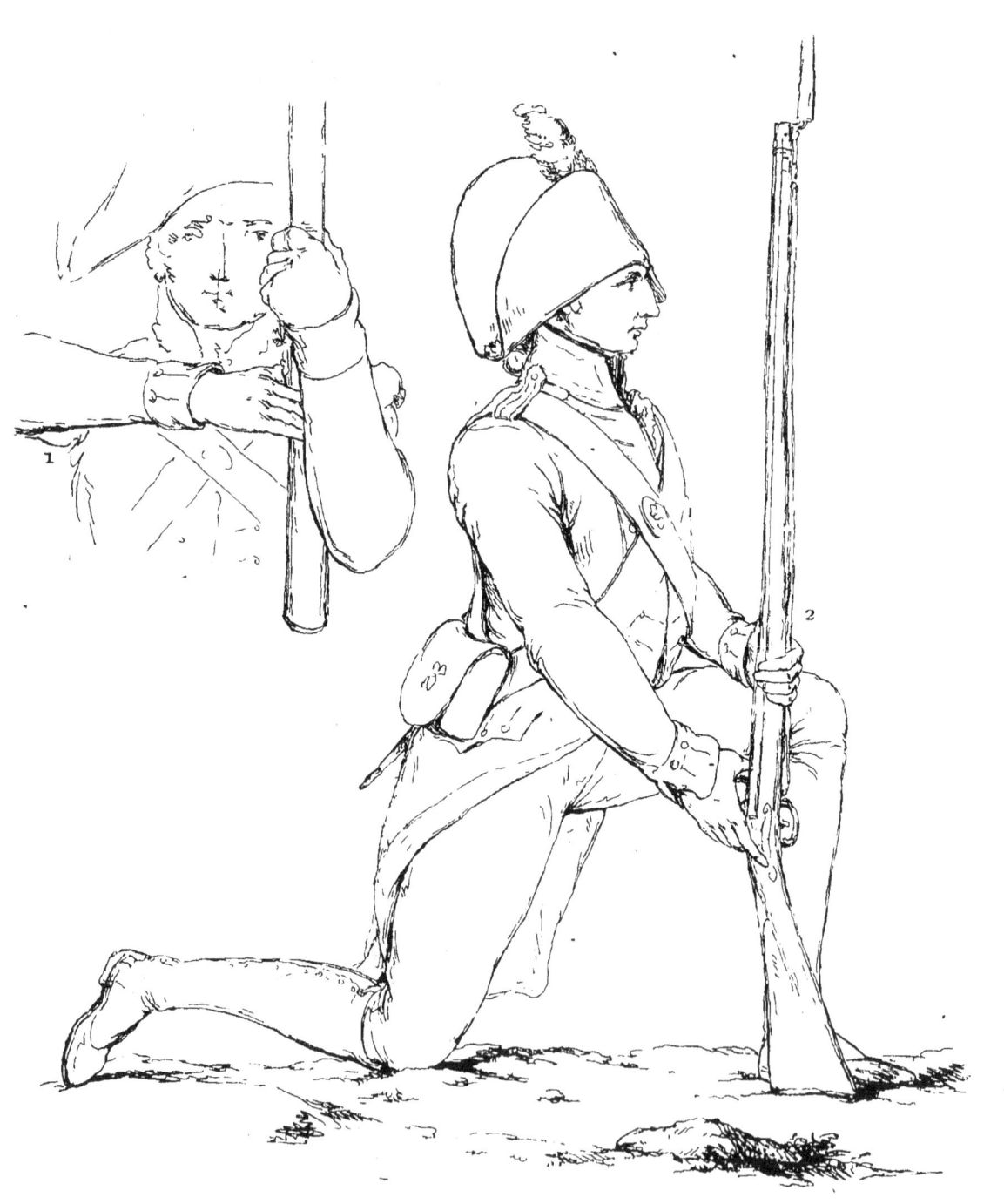

Published as the Act directs Aug.st 30.th 1798 at Egerton's Military Library Whitehall

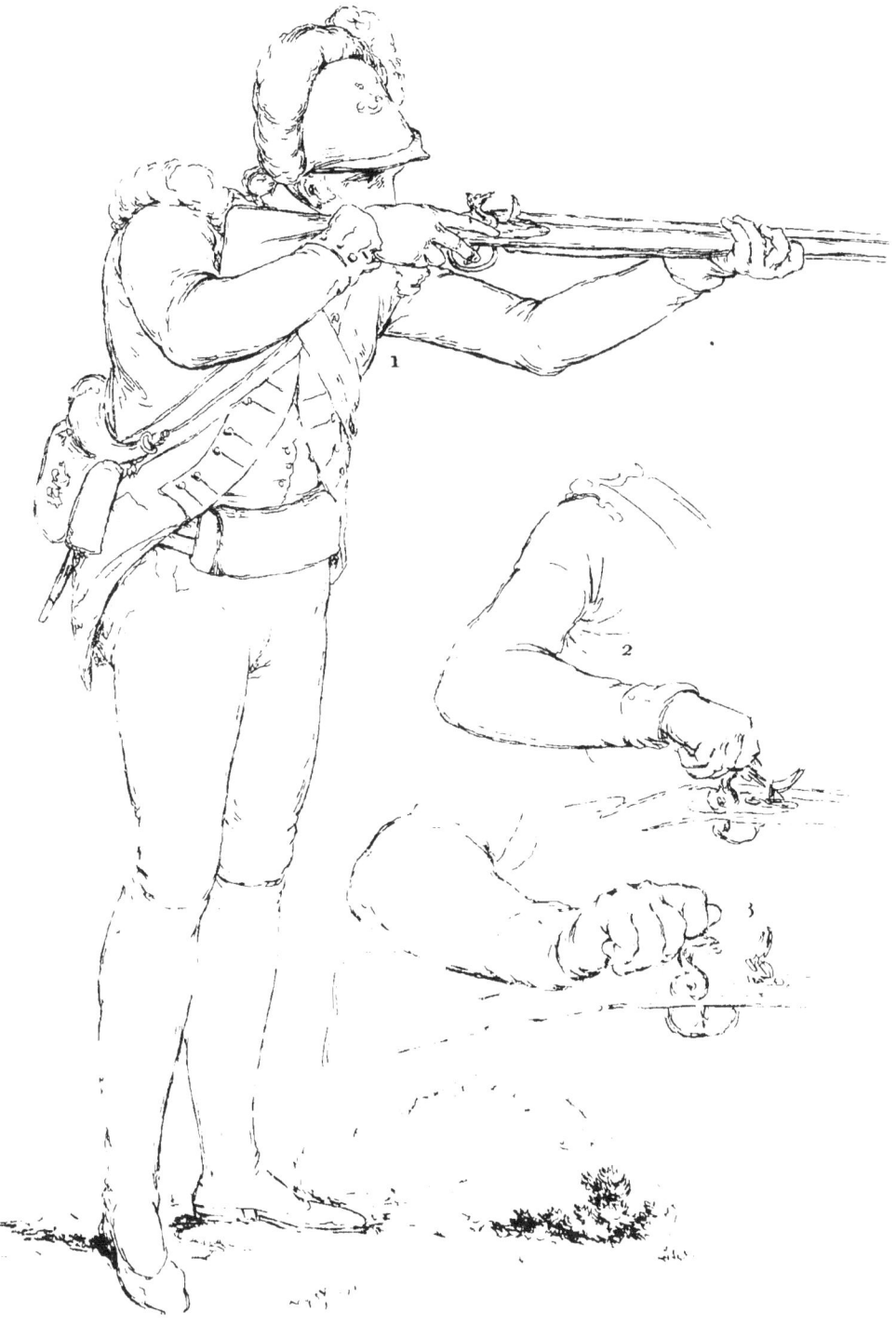

1

2

Published as the Act directs, Aug.st 10th, 1798 at Egert.ns Military Lib.y   Whitehall

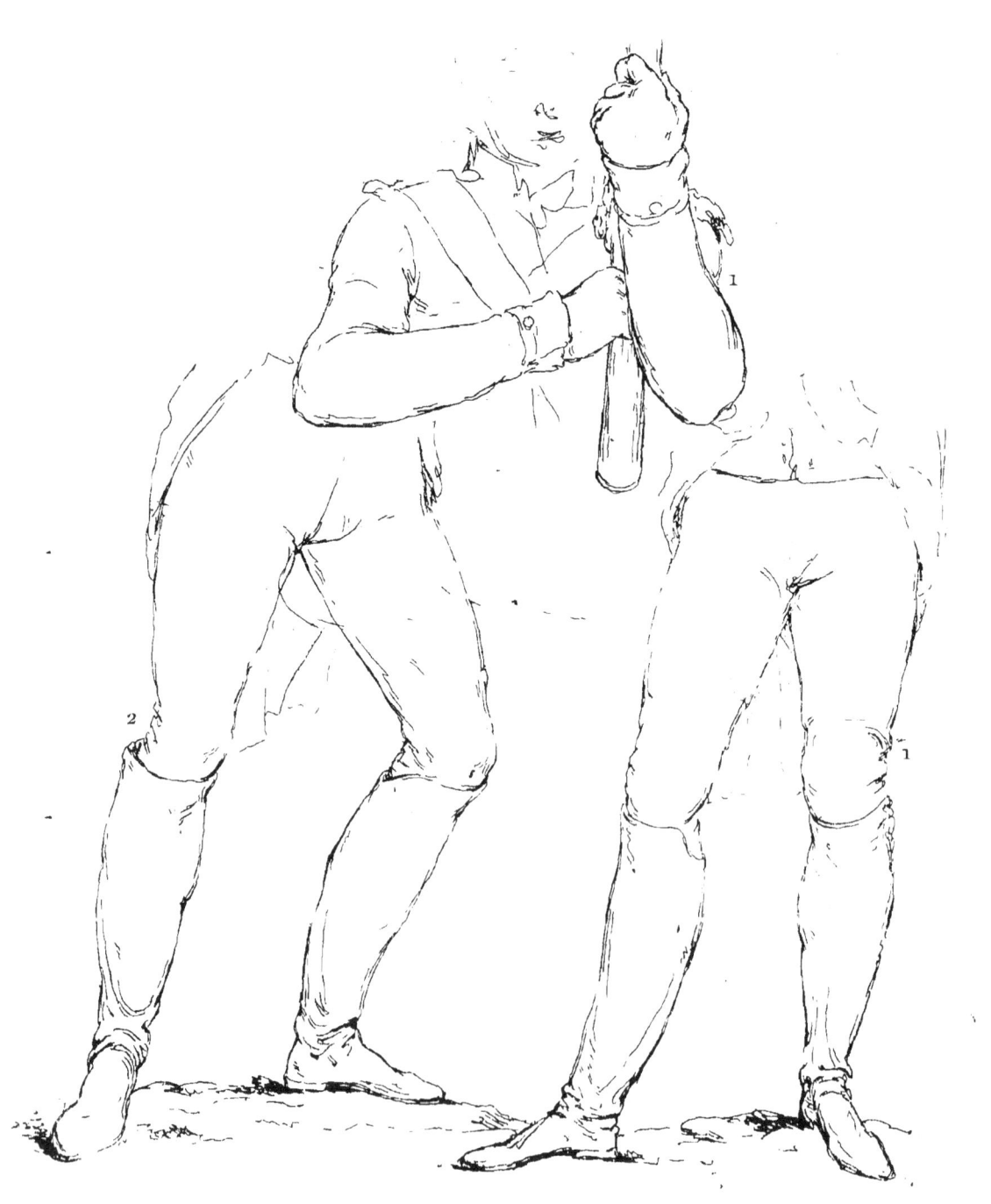

Published as the Act directs, Aug.st 10.th 1798 at Egertons Military Library Whitehall

PLATE XXII

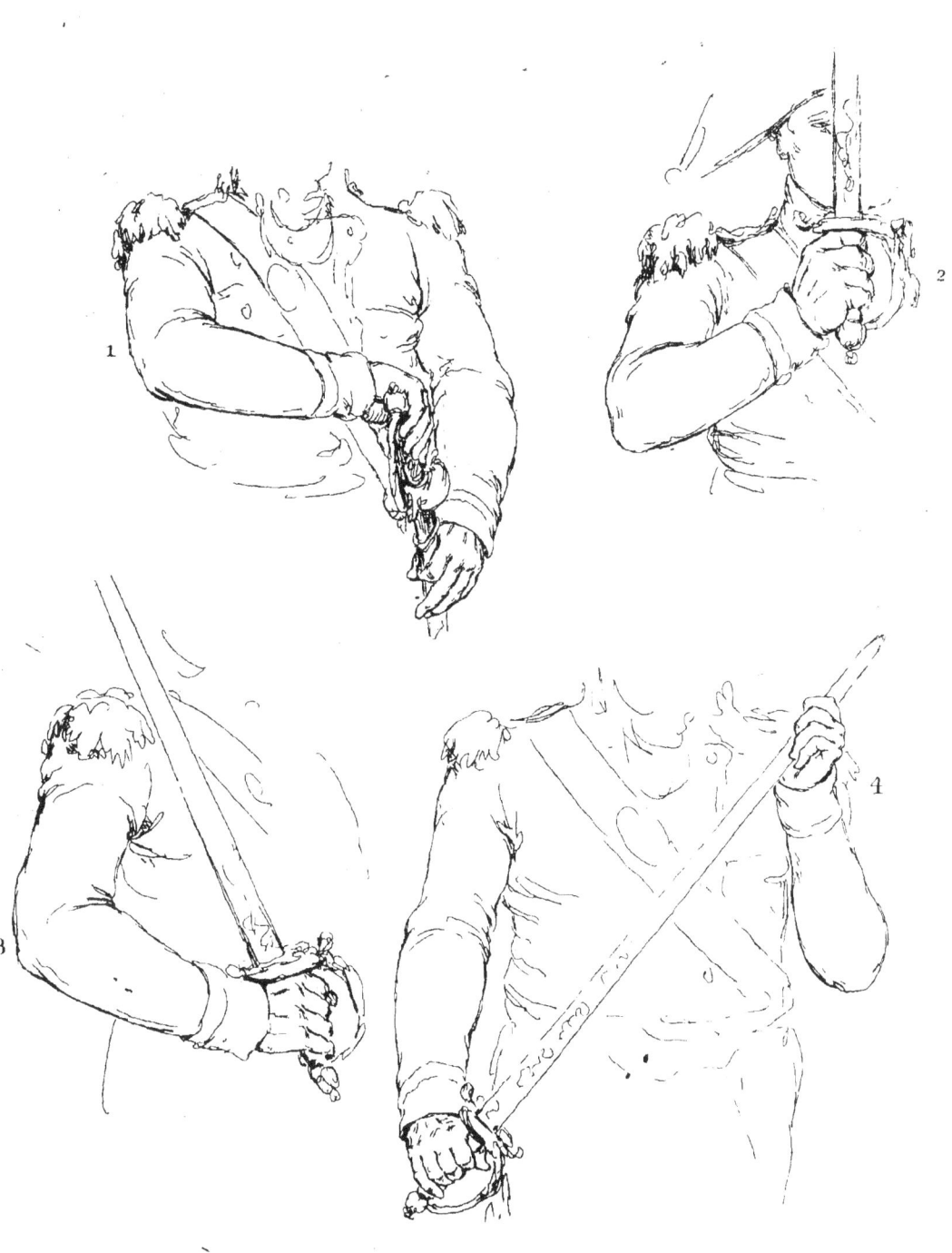

Published as the Act directs Augᵗ 30ᵗʰ 1798 at Egertons Military Library Whitehall

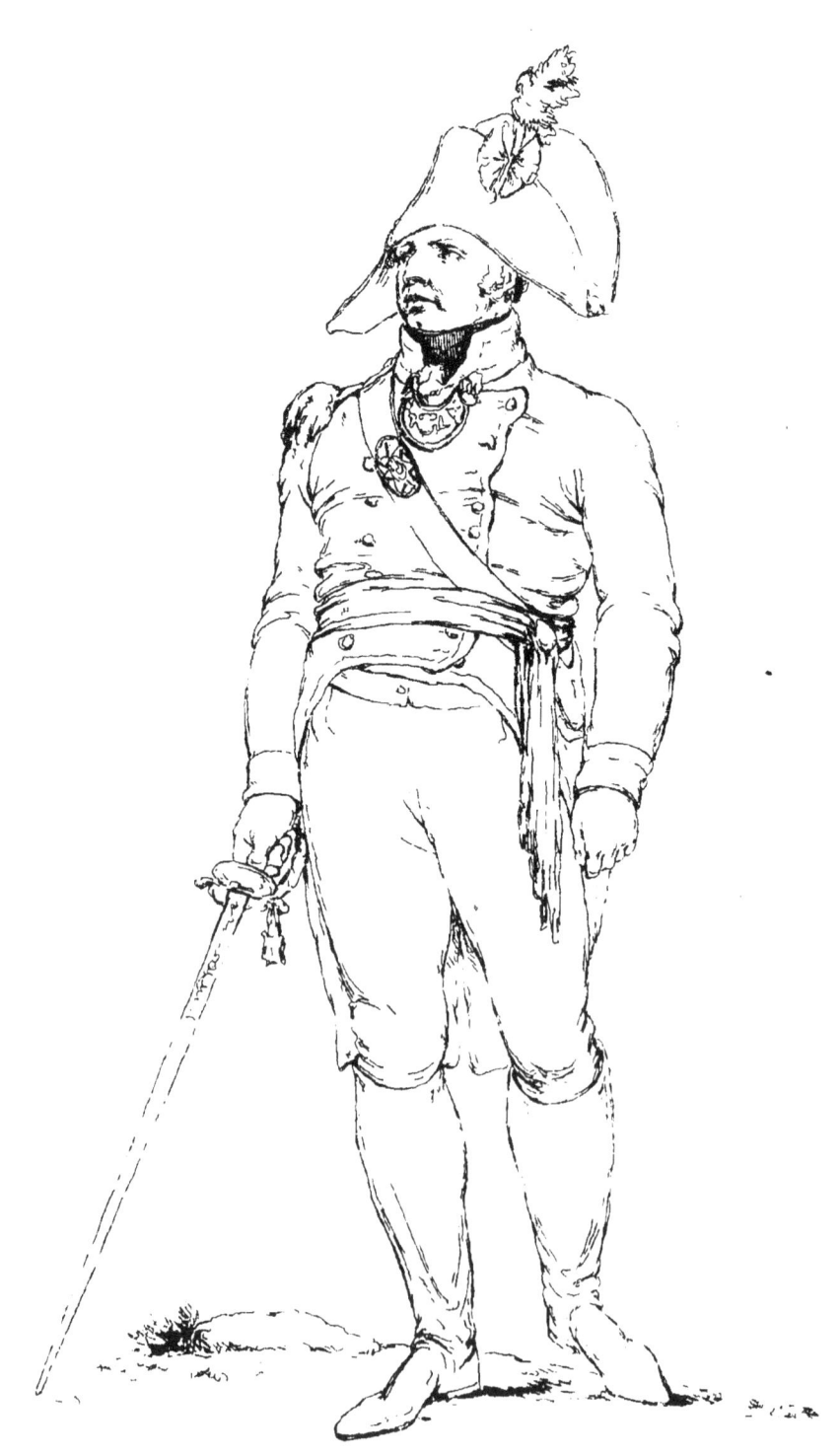

Published as the Act directs Aug.ᵗ 14ᵗʰ 1798 at R. Pollards Side ... ... W. ... ...

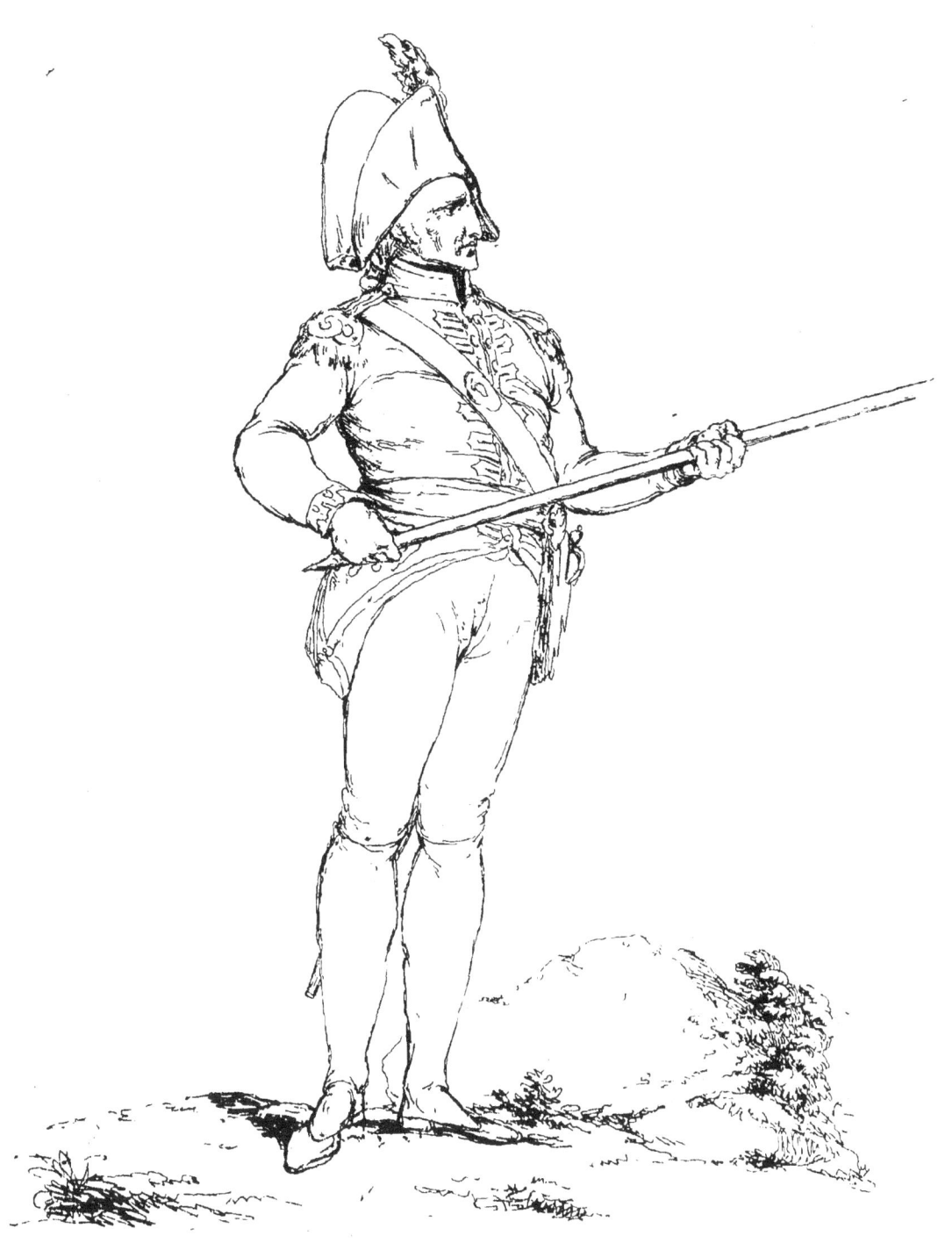

Published as the Act directs Aug.st 30.th 1798 at Egertons Military Library Whitehall

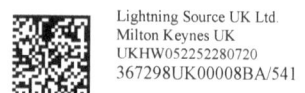

Lightning Source UK Ltd.
Milton Keynes UK
UKHW052252280720
367298UK00008BA/541

9 781140 857884